CONCISE
DICTIONARY OF
SYNONYMS
ANTONYMS

Useful Guide for Aspirants of IAS, CAT, GMAT, GRE, Civil Services, IELTS, TOEFL & Other Examinations

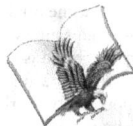

V&S PUBLISHERS

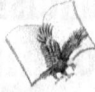

Published by:

V&S PUBLISHERS

F-2/16, Ansari road, Daryaganj, New Delhi-110002
☎ 23240026, 23240027 • *Fax:* 011-23240028
Email: info@vspublishers.com • *Website:* www.vspublishers.com

Regional Office : Hyderabad
5-1-707/1, Brij Bhawan (Beside Central Bank of India Lane)
Bank Street, Koti, Hyderabad - 500 095
☎ 040-24737290
E-mail: vspublishershyd@gmail.com

Branch Office : Mumbai
Jaywant Industrial Estate, 1st Floor–108, Tardeo Road
Opposite Sobo Central Mall, Mumbai – 400 034
☎ 022-23510736
E-mail: vspublishersmum@gmail.com

BUY OUR BOOKS FROM: AMAZON FLIPKART

© **Copyright:** V&S PUBLISHERS
ISBN 978-93-505716–6–8

Edition 2020

DISCLAIMER

While every attempt has been made to provide accurate and timely information in this book, neither the author nor the publisher assumes any responsibility for errors, unintended omissions or commissions detected therein. The author and publisher make no representation or warranty with respect to the comprehensiveness or completeness of the contents provided.

All matters included have been simplified under professional guidance for general information only without any warranty for applicability on an individual. Any mention of an organization or a website in the book by way of citation or as a source of additional information doesn't imply the endorsement of the content either by the author or the publisher. It is possible that websites cited may have changed or removed between the time of editing and publishing the book.

Results from using the expert opinion in this book will be totally dependent on individual circumstances and factors beyond the control of the author and the publisher.

It makes sense to elicit advice from well informed sources before implementing the ideas given in the book. The reader assumes full responsibility for the consequences arising out from reading this book. For proper guidance, it is advisable to read the book under the watchful eyes of parents/guardian. The purchaser of this book assumes all responsibility for the use of given materials and information. The copyright of the entire content of this book rests with the author/publisher. Any infringement/ transmission of the cover design, text or illustrations, in any form, by any means, by any entity will invite legal action and be responsible for consequences thereon.

Publisher's Note

Considering the grand success of the **EXC-EL Series (Excellence in English Language Series)** which consists of four books - *English Vocabulary Made Easy, English Grammar & Usage, Spoken English and Improve Your Vocabulary*, we have come up with a number of **English Dictionaries** pertaining to **Proverbs, Idioms, Phrases, Similes and Metaphors.** This book, *Concise Dictionary of Synonyms and Antonyms* is an addition to this series. Besides the above, V&S Publishers has also come out with a whole lot of **Concise Dictionaries of Physics, Chemistry, Biology, Science, Mathematics, Economics, Commerce, Management and Computers-** both in English and Hindi.

Being aware that our existence as a publishing house depends solely upon fulfilling our readers' expectations and continued patronage, we decided to come out with something that can add a spark to any conversation, while making it appear interesting.

This *Combined and Concise Dictionary of Synonyms Antonyms* has five distinct sections: A list of commonly used Antonyms or Opposite Words, A list of popular Synonyms or words with similar meanings, Multiple Choice Questions (MCQs) related to Antonyms, MCQs related to Synonyms and a section containing the Answers of both the MCQs.

English, as we all know is an immensely popular, attractive, articulate, rich and diverse language, but a versatile knowledge of Words and their Meanings (Synonyms) and Words and their Opposites (Antonyms) are a must for readers of all ages who are keen to master the language by improving their Word Power and Vocabulary, particularly the student section in various schools and colleges.

Hence, this book has been aimed primarily to enhance and enrich the English vocabulary of our esteemed readers and to help the student faculty academically to speak as well as write fluent, error-free and excellent English.

'To err is human', and hence, we apologise if any errors have inadvertently crept in the book; and would be glad to rectify them with your valuable suggestions, views and comments, thus improving the content and quality of future editions.

SYNONYMS

SYNONYMS

The word, 'synonym' has been derived from the Greek word, *syn (with)* and *onoma (name). Synonyms are words or expressions with the same or nearly the same meanings.* The words may be used as figurative or symbolic substitutes as they have identical meanings. They can be any parts of speech, such as *nouns, verbs, adjectives, adverbs* or *prepositions. A word can have more than one synonym.*

Synonyms are very useful. There are times when one avoids repeating the same words over and over again, and it becomes hard to think of an alternative word. A person well equipped with synonyms might not face these problems as the words come handy.

For example:

Synonyms for 'hardworking' are 'diligent', 'determined'. 'industrious' and 'enterprising'. Similarly, synonyms for 'beautiful' are pretty, attractive, stunning and lovely and the synonyms for' kind' are considerate, thoughtful, gracious, amiable, etc.

A

Abeyance *(noun)*–A state of temporary disuse or suspension
- Suspension *(noun)*
- Remission *(noun)*
- Reserve *(noun)*
- Dormant *(adjective)*

Abase *(verb)* –Deprive of self-esteem, confidence
- Belittle *(verb)*
- Debase *(verb)*
- Diminish *(verb)*
- Degrade *(verb)*

Abhor *(verb)* –Regard with contempt or disgust
- Despise *(verb)*
- Detest *(verb)*
- Loathe *(verb)*
- Scorn *(verb)*

Abject *(adjective)*–Hopeless and downtrodden
- Wretched *(adjective)*
- Deplorable *(adjective)*
- Base *(adjective)*
- Dejected *(adjective)*

Abduct *(verb)* –Take by force and without permission
- Kidnap *(verb)*
- Grab *(verb)*
- Seize *(verb)*
- Snatch *(verb)*

Abomination *(noun)*–A thing that causes disgust or loathing
- Atrocity *(noun)*
- Monstrocity *(noun)*
- Torment *(noun)*
- Horror *(noun)*

Ablaze *(adjective)*–Burning fiercely
- Alight *(verb)*
- Aflame *(adjective)*
- Flaming *(adjective)*
- Blazing *(adjective)*

Abrasive *(adjective)*–Irritating in manner
- Cutting *(adjective)*
- Caustic *(adjective)*
- Annoying *(adjective)*
- Nasty *(adjective)*

Abstain *(verb)* –Hold back from doing
- Quit *(verb)*
- Refuse *(verb)*
- Pass *(verb)*
- Cease *(verb)*

Abstract *(adjective)*–Conceptual, theoretical
- Complex *(adjective)*
- Unreal *(adjective)*
- Deep *(adjective)*
- Ideal *(adjective)*

Abundant *(adjective)*–Plentiful, large in number
    Ample *(adjective)*
    Heavy *(adjective)*
    Rich *(adjective)*
    Sufficient *(adjective)*

Abstemious *(adjective)*–Indulging only very moderately in something, especially food and drink.
    Abstinent *(adjective)*
    Austere *(adjective)*
    Moderate *(adjective)*
    Restrained *(adjective)*

Abstruse *(adjective)*–Difficult to understand; obscure.
    Difficult *(adjective)*
    Puzzling *(adjective)*
    Cryptic *(adjective)*
    Incomprehensible *(adjective)*

Abysmal *(adjective)*–Great extent; immeasurable
    Bottomless *(adjective)*
    Endless *(adjective)*
    Complete *(adjective)*
    Boundless *(adjective)*

Accept *(verb)* –Receive something given physically
    Get *(verb)*
    Take *(verb)*
    Welcome *(verb)*
    Acquire *(verb)*

Accentuate *(verb)* –Focus attention on
    Highlight *(verb)*
    Emphasize *(verb)*
    Underline *(verb)*
    Underscore *(verb)*

Accomplice *(noun)*–Helper, especially in committing a crime
    Aide *(noun)*
    Associate *(noun)*
    Ally *(noun)*
    Partner *(noun)*

Aching *(adjective)*–Painful
    Hurting *(adjective)*
    Sore *(adjective)*
    Throbbing *(adjective)*
    Nagging *(adjective)*

Acrimonious *(adjective)*–Nasty in behaviour, speech
    Angry *(adjective)*
    Cutting *(adjective)*
    Sarcastic *(adjective)*
    Belligerent *(adjective)*

Acute *(adjective)*–Deeply perceptive
    Keen *(adjective)*
    Astute *(adjective)*
    Sharp *(adjective)*
    Subtle *(adjective)*

Accoutre *(verb)* –Clothe or equip in something noticeable or impressive.
    Decorate *(verb)*
    Embellish *(verb)*
    Furnish *(verb)*
    Outfit *(verb)*

Accord *(noun)*–An official agreement or treaty
    Pact *(noun)*
    Treaty *(noun)*
    Settlement *(noun)*
    Concord *(noun)*

Accost *(verb)* –Approach for conversation or solicitation
Annoy *(verb)*
Brace *(verb)*
Confront *(verb)*
Entice *(verb)*

Acclivity *(noun)*–An upward slope
Elevation *(noun)*
Hill *(noun)*
Rise *(noun)*
Upgrade *(noun)*

Acme *(noun)*–The point at which something is at its best or most highly developed
Climax *(noun)*
Culmination *(noun)*
Zenith *(noun)*
Summit *(noun)*

Acquit *(verb)* –Announce removal of blame
Vindicate *(verb)*
Excuse *(verb)*
Absolve *(verb)*
Liberate *(verb)*

Acumen *(noun)*–Ability to understand and reason
Intellect *(noun)*
Wisdom *(noun)*
Insight *(noun)*
Brilliance *(noun)*

Adapt *(verb)* –Adjust to a different situation or condition
Modify *(verb)*
Alter *(verb)*
Convert *(verb)*
Transform *(verb)*

Adamant *(adjective)*–Unyielding
Determined *(adjective)*
Insistent *(adjective)*
Resolute *(adjective)*
Rigid *(adjective)*

Admonish *(verb)* –Warn, strongly criricize
Advise *(verb)*
Berate *(verb)*
Censure *(verb)*
Rebuke *(verb)*

Adorn *(verb)* –Decorate
Eautify *(verb)*
Grace *(verb)*
Enrich *(verb)*
Embellish *(verb)*

Adroit *(adjective)*–Very able or skilled
Adept *(adjective)*
Clever *(adjective)*
Handy *(adjective)*
Artful *(adjective)*

Aesthetic *(adjective)*–Beautiful
Artistic *(adjective)*
Creative *(adjective)*
Artful *(adjective)*
Inventive *(adjective)*

Affable *(adjective)*–Friendly
Pleasant *(adjective)*
Amiable *(adjective)*
Gracious *(adjective)*
Benign *(adjective)*

Affinity *(noun)*–Liking or inclination towards something
Affection *(noun)*
Sympathy *(noun)*
Closeness *(noun)*
Fondness *(noun)*

Affliction *(noun)*–Hurt condition; something that causes hurt
Disease *(noun)*
Calamity *(noun)*
Hardship *(noun)*
Disorder *(noun)*

Affluent *(adjective)*–Wealthy
Moneyed *(adjective)*
Upscale *(adjective)*
Flush *(adjective)*
Rich *(adjective)*

Adulation *(noun)*–Overenthusiastic praise
Applause *(noun)*
Flattery *(noun)*
Worship *(noun)*
Sycophancy *(noun)*

Advocacy *(noun)*–Support for an idea or cause
Backing *(noun)*
Assistance *(noun)*
Promotion *(noun)*
Justification *(noun)*

Adversity *(noun)*–Bad luck, situation
Calamity *(noun)*
Mishap *(noun)*
Disaster *(noun)*
Hardship *(noun)*

Adjoin *(verb)*–Be next to
Connect *(verb)*
Join *(verb)*
Touch *(verb)*
Verge *(verb)*

Adhere *(verb)*–Conform to or follow rules exactly
Comply *(verb)*
Heed *(verb)*

Obey *(verb)*
Follow *(verb)*

Adjourn *(verb)*–Stop a proceeding
Defer *(verb)*
Delay *(verb)*
Discontinue *(verb)*
Harmony *(verb)*

Adjudge *(verb)*–Judge
Adjudicate *(verb)*
Consider *(verb)*
Decide *(verb)*
Determine *(verb)*

Adept *(adjective)*–Very able
Accomplished *(noun)*– *(adjective)*
Capable *(adjective)*
Skilled *(adjective)*
Expert *(adjective)*

Adjust *(verb)*–Become or make prepared, adapted
Conform *(verb)*
Alter *(verb)*
Order *(verb)*
accomodate *(verb)*

Advice *(noun)*–Recommendation
Aid *(noun)*
Opinion *(noun)*
Help *(noun)*
Guidance *(noun)*

Aficionado *(noun)*–A person who is very knowledgeable and enthusiastic about an activity, subject, or pastime
Connoisseur *(noun)*
Expert *(adjective)*
Authority *(noun)*
Fan *(noun)*

Affirm *(verb)*–Declare the truth of something
Confirm *(verb)*

Declare *(verb)*
Insist *(verb)*
Assert *(verb)*

Affect *(verb)* –Influence, affect emotionally
  Disturb *(verb)*
  Alter *(verb)*
  Change *(verb)*
  Interest *(verb)*

Agile *(adjective)*–Physically or mentally nimble, deft
  Rapid *(adjective)*
  Quick *(adjective)*
  Mercurial *(adjective)*
  Brisk *(adjective)*

Akimbo *(adverb)* –With hands on the hips and elbows turned outwards
  Jagged *(adjective)*
  Skewed *(verb)*
  Oblique *(adjective)*
  Slanted *(adjective)*

Alacrity *(noun)*–Brisk and cheerful readiness
  Eagerness *(noun)*
  Willingness *(noun)*
  Readiness *(noun)*
  Zeal *(noun)*

Alcove *(noun)*–A recess in the wall of a room or garden
  Niche *(noun)*
  Nook *(noun)*
  Bay *(noun)*
  Corner *(noun)*

Ale *(noun)*–Any beer other than lager, stout or porter.
  Brew *(noun)*
  Malt *(noun)*

Beer *(noun)*
Hops *(noun)*

Alight *(verb)* –Descend from a trains, bus or other form of transport
  Dismount *(verb)*
  Disembark *(verb)*
  Step off *(verb)*
  Exit *(verb)*

Alienate *(verb)* –Cause unfriendliness, hostility
  Disaffect *(verb)*
  Separate *(verb)*
  Divide *(verb)*
  Estrange *(verb)*

Allege *(verb)* –Assert; claim
  Charge *(verb)*
  Recount *(verb)*
  Recite *(verb)*
  Affirm *(verb)*

Allegiance *(noun)*–Loyalty
  Adherence *(noun)*
  Faithfulness *(noun)*
  Obedience *(noun)*
  Devotion *(noun)*

Alleviate *(verb)* –Relieve; lessen
  Ease *(verb)*
  Allay *(verb)*
  Pacify *(verb)*
  Mollify *(verb)*

Allude *(verb)* –Hint at
  Advert *(verb)*
  Insinuate *(verb)*
  Point *(verb)*
  Suggest *(verb)*

Altruistic *(adjective)*–Unselfish
  Charitable *(adjective)*
  Humanitarian *(adjective)*

benevolent *(adjective)*
Generous *(adjective)*

Aloof *(adjective)*–Remote
Detached *(adjective)*
Distant *(adjective)*
Haughty *(adjective)*
Indifferent *(adjective)*

Aloft *(adjective and adverb)* –Up in or into the air; overhead
Upwards *(adverb)*
Skyward *(adjective)*
High up *(adjective)*
Up above *(adjective)*

Allusion *(noun)*–An expression designed to call something to mind without mentioning it explicitly; an indirect or passing reference
Implication *(noun)*
Insinuation *(noun)*
Hint at *(verb)*
Citation of *(verb)*

Amaze *(verb)* –Surprise
Perplex *(verb)*
Bewilder *(verb)*
Daze *(verb)*
Impress *(verb)*

Ambiguous *(adjective)*–Having more than one meaning
Enigmatic *(adjective)*
Opaque *(adjective)*
Obscure *(adjective)*
Vague *(adjective)*

Amiable *(adjective)*–Friendly, agreeable
Affable *(adjective)*
Lovable *(adjective)*
Cozy *(adjective)*
Cordial *(adjective)*

Ambivalent *(adjective)*–Conflicting
Contradictory *(adjective)*
Uncertain *(adjective)*
Fluctuating *(adjective)*
Uncertain *(adjective)*

Ample *(adjective)*–More than necessary, sufficient
Abundant *(adjective)*
Spacious *(adjective)*
Enough *(adjective)*
Plenty *(adjective)*

Animosity *(noun)*–Extreme dislike, hatred
Acrimony *(noun)*
Bitterness *(noun)*
Malice *(noun)*
Antipathy *(noun)*

Annihilate *(verb)* –Destroy completely
Crush *(verb)*
decimate *(verb)*
Demolish *(verb)*
Eradicate *(verb)*

Anomaly *(noun)*–Deviation from normal, usual
Aberration *(noun)*
Deviation *(noun)*
Oddity *(noun)*
Rarity *(noun)*

Anonymous *(adjective)*–Unknown, usually by choice
Unidentified *(adjective)*
Unacknowledged *(adjective)*
Secret *(adjective)*
Unsigned *(adjective)*

Apex *(noun)*–Top, high point
Climax *(noun)*
Pinnacle *(noun)*

Max *(noun)*
Culmination *(noun)*

Approbation *(noun)*–Approval or praise
Approval *(noun)*
Acceptance *(noun)*
Endorsement *(noun)*
Appreciation *(noun)*

Aquiline *(adjective)*–Like an eagle
Beaked *(adjective)*
Prominent *(adjective)*
Eaglelike *(adjective)*
Roman-nosed *(adjective)*

Ambivalence *(noun)*–The state of having mixed feelings or contradictory ideas about something or someone.
Uncertainty *(noun)*
Doubt *(noun)*
Irresolution *(noun)*
Vacillation *(noun)*

Ambrosia *(noun)*–The food of the gods
Delicacy *(noun)*
Nectar *(noun)*
Heavenly food *(noun)*
Immortal food *(noun)*

Ameliorate *(verb)* –Make *(something bad or unsatisfactory)* better
Alleviate *(verb)*
Lighten *(verb)*
Improve *(verb)*
Amend *(verb)*

Anachronism *(noun)*– A thing belonging or appropriate to a period other than that in which it exists, especially a thing that is conspicu-
ously old-fashioned
Misplacement *(noun)*
Prolepsis *(noun)*
Chronological error *(noun)*
Misdate *(noun)*

Antics *(noun)*–Foolish, outrageous or amusing behaviour
Capers *(noun)*
Pranks *(noun)*
Larks *(noun)*
Escapades *(noun)*

Annex *(noun)*–A building joined to or associated with a main building, providing additional space or accommodation
Addendum *(noun)*
Addition *(noun)*
Supplement *(noun)*
Wing *(noun)*

Annihilate *(verb)* –Destroy completely
Obliterate *(verb)*
Exterminate *(verb)*
Eliminate *(verb)*
Eradicate *(verb)*

Aplomb *(noun)*–Self-confidence or assurance, especially when in a demanding situation
Poise *(noun)*
Composure *(noun)*
Sangfroid *(noun)*
Nonchalance *(noun)*

Aptitude *(noun)*–Inclination
Disposition *(noun)*
Drift *(noun)*
Bent *(noun)*
Leaning *(noun)*

Arbitrary *(adjective)*–Whimsical, chance
    Irresponsible *(adjective)*
    Capricious *(adjective)*
    Fanciful *(adjective)*
    Wayward *(adjective)*

Arcane *(adjective)*–Hidden, secret
    Esoteric *(adjective)*
    Mystic *(adjective)*
    Occult *(adjective)*
    Mysterious *(adjective)*

Archaic *(adjective)*–Very old
    Ancient *(adjective)*
    Old-fashioned *(adjective)*
    Antique *(adjective)*
    Bygone *(adjective)*

Archetype *(noun)*–Typical example
    Form *(noun)*
    Original *(noun)*
    Prototype *(noun)*
    Model *(noun)*

Ardent *(adjective)*–Very enthusiastic
    Avid *(adjective)*
    Fervent *(adjective)*
    Fierce *(adjective)*
    Zealous *(adjective)*

Arduous *(adjective)*–Difficult, hard to endure
    Uphill *(adjective)*
    Exhausting *(adjective)*
    Painful *(adjective)*
    Punishing *(adjective)*

Aristocratic *(adjective)*–Priviledged, elegant
    Noble *(adjective)*
    Dignified *(adjective)*
    Patrician *(adjective)*
    Elite *(adjective)*

Artifice *(noun)*–Hoax; clever act
    Gimmick *(noun)*
    Scam *(noun)*
    Expedient *(noun)*
    Device *(noun)*

Ascetic *(adjective)*–Self-denying
    Austere *(adjective)*
    Abstinent *(adjective)*
    Abstaining *(adjective)*
    Disciplined *(adjective)*

Aspire *(verb)* –Aim, hope
    Pursue *(verb)*
    Desire *(verb)*
    Crave *(verb)*
    Yearn *(verb)*

Atone *(verb)*–Compensate, make amends for former misdoing
    Redeem *(verb)*
    Pay *(verb)*
    Answer *(verb)*
    Apologise *(verb)*

Attest *(verb)* –Affirm, vouch for
    Authenticate *(verb)*
    Announce *(verb)*
    Display *(verb)*
    Testify *(verb)*

Attire *(noun)*–Clothing
    Apparel *(noun)*
    Clothes *(noun)*
    Garb *(noun)*
    Costume *(noun)*

Attribute *(noun)*–Feature
    Aspect *(noun)*
    Facet *(noun)*
    Quality *(noun)*
    Trait *(noun)*

Audacious *(adjective)*–Reckless, daring
- Foolhardy *(adjective)*
- Gutty *(adjective)*
- Undaunted *(adjective)*
- Cheeky *(adjective)*

Audible *(adjective)*–Able to be heard
- Deafening *(adjective)*
- Loud *(adjective)*
- Clear *(adjective)*
- Distinct (*adjective*)

Augment *(verb)*–Make greater, improve
- Develop *(verb)*
- Heighten *(verb)*
- Compound *(verb)*
- Progress *(verb)*

Augur *(noun)*–Predictor
- Herald *(noun)*
- Prophet *(noun)*
- Seer *(noun)*
- Forecast *(noun)*

Austere *(adjective)*–Severe in manner
- Stringent *(adjective)*
- Stern *(adjective)*
- Harsh *(adjective)*
- Rigid (*adjective*)

Authentic *(adjective)*–Real, genuine
- Accurate *(adjective)*
- Reliable *(adjective)*
- Credible *(adjective)*
- Convincing (*adjective*)

Avarice *(noun)*–Extreme greed
- Frugality *(noun)*
- Avidity *(noun)*
- Greediness *(noun)*
- Thrift *(noun)*

Apparition *(noun)*–A ghost or ghostlike image of a person
- Phantom *(noun)*
- Spectre *(noun)*
- Spirit *(noun)*
- Wraith *(noun)*

Artlessly *(adverb)*–In a crude and unskilled manner
- Easily *(adverb)*
- Simply *(adverb)*
- Casually *(adverb)*
- Impulsively *(adverb)*

Arbitration *(noun)*–The use of an arbitrator to settle a dispute
- Mediation *(noun)*
- Negotiation *(noun)*
- Conciliation *(noun)*
- Intervention *(noun)*

Ark *(noun)*–A place of protection or security; *(in the Bible)* the large boat built by Noah
- Barge *(noun)*
- Refuge *(noun)*
- Retreat *(noun)*
- Ship *(noun)*
- Vessel *(noun)*

Arson *(verb)*–The criminal act of deliberately setting fire to property
- Incendiarism *(noun)*
- Pyromania *(noun)*
- Firebombing *(noun)*
- Fire-raising *(noun)*

Askance *(adverb)*–With an attitude or look of suspicion or disapproval
- Suspiciously *(adverb)*
- Skeptically *(adverb)*
- Doubtfully *(adverb)*
- Mistrustfully *(adverb)*

Astute *(adjective)*–Perceptive
  Crafty *(adjective)*
  Foxy *(adjective)*
  Savvy *(adjective)*
  Intelligent *(adjective)*

Astound *(verb)* –Amaze
  Astonish *(verb)*
  Shock *(verb)*
  Stagger *(verb)*

August *(adjective)*–Respected and impressive
  Distinguished *(adjective)*
  Eminent *(adjective)*
  Illustrious *(adjective)*
  Acclaimed *(adjective)*

Arraign *(verb)* –Call or bring someone before a court to answer a criminal charge
  Indict *(verb)*
  Prosecute *(verb)*
  Take to court *(verb)*
  Summons *(noun)*

Arrears *(noun)*–Money that is owed and should have been paid earlier
  Outstanding payment *(noun)*
  Debt *(noun)*
  Dues *(noun)*
  Liabilities *(noun)*

Ashen *(adjective)*–Very pale with shock, fear or illness
  Wan *(adjective)*
  Colourless *(adjective)*
  Sallow *(adjective)*
  Waxen *(adjective)*

Asyndeton *(noun)*–The omission or absence of a conjunction between parts of a sentence
  Allusion *(noun)*
  Manner of speaking *(noun)*
  Turn of phrase *(noun)*
  That is not meant *(noun)*

Avenge *(verb)* –Retaliate
  Vindicate *(verb)*
  Repay (*verb*)
  Punish (*verb*)
  Requite *(verb)*

Aversion *(noun)*–Dislike; opposition
  Distaste *(noun)*
  Antipathy *(noun)*
  Allergy *(noun)*
  Hatred *(noun)*

Avid *(adjective)*–Enthusiastic
  Voracious *(adjective)*
  Eager (*adjective*)
  Ardent *(adjective)*
  Ravenous *(adjective)*

Awe *(noun)*–Amazement
  Admiration (*noun*)
  Awe (*noun*)
  Esteem (*noun*)
  Wonder (*noun*)

Abridge *(verb)* –Shorten
  Curtail *(verb)*
  Lessen *(verb)*
  Abbreviate *(verb)*
  Downsize *(verb)*

Adrift *(adverb)* –floating out of control
  Afloat *(adverb)*
  Unmoored (*adverb*)
  Loose *(adverb)*
  Drifting *(adverb)*

Abode *(noun)*–Building or place where one resides
- Home *(noun)*
- Sanctuary *(noun)*
- Domicile *(noun)*
- Address *(noun)*

Accolade *(noun)*–Strong praise, recognition of achievement
- Distinction *(noun)*

- Approval *(noun)*
- Badge *(noun)*
- Honor *(noun)*

Ascent *(noun)*–Upward movement
- Climb *(noun)*
- Rise *(noun)*
- Lift *(noun)*
- Mounting *(noun)*

B

Baffle *(verb)* –Perplex
   Mystify *(verb)*
   Puzzle *(verb)*
   Stun *(verb)*
   Bewilder *(verb)*

Avouch *(verb)* –Assert
   Admit *(verb)*
   Affirm *(verb)*
   Avow *(verb)*
   maintain *(verb)*

Avow *(verb)* –Assert or confess openly
   Declare *(verb)*
   State *(verb)*
   Attest *(verb)*
   Swear *(verb)*

Bacchanal *(noun)*–A wild and drunken celebration
   Carnival *(noun)*
   Feast *(noun)*
   Frolic *(noun)*
   Party *(noun)*

Baleful *(adjective)*–Menacing
   Harmful *(adjective)*
   Deadly *(adjective)*
   Evil *(adjective)*
   Sinister *(adjective)*

Balk *(verb)* –Stop short
   Flinch *(verb)*
   Resist *(verb)*
   Recoil *(verb)*
   Refuse *(verb)*

Ban *(noun)*–Official forbiddance
   Boycott *(noun)*
   Refusal *(noun)*
   Stoppage *(noun)*
   Prohibition *(noun)*

Banish *(verb)* –Expel from place or situation
   Dismiss *(verb)*
   Dispel *(verb)*
   Exile *(verb)*
   Deport *(verb)*

Barbaric *(adjective)*–Crude, savage
   Cruel *(adjective)*
   Inhuman *(adjective)*
   Rough *(adjective)*
   Boorish *(adjective)*

Barrage *(noun)*–Weapon fire
   Blast *(noun)*
   Shower *(noun)*
   Hail *(noun)*
   Storm *(noun)*

Barren *(adjective)*–Unable to support growth
   Desolate *(adjective)*
   Arid *(adjective)*
   Empty *(adjective)*
   Desert *(adjective)*

Bastion *(noun)*–Support; fortified place
    Fortress *(noun)*
    Citadel *(noun)*
    Stronghold *(noun)*
    Support *(noun)*

Befuddle *(verb)* –Confuse
    Dumbfound *(verb)*
    Daze *(verb)*
    Puzzle *(verb)*
    Distract *(verb)*

Beguile *(verb)* –Fool
    Deceive *(verb)*
    Delude *(verb)*
    Mislead *(verb)*
    Betray *(verb)*

Bandeau *(noun)*–A narrow band worn round the head to hold the hair in position
    Scarf *(noun)*
    Snood *(noun)*
    Ribbon *(noun)*
    Sash *(noun)*

Bawdy *(adjective)*–Humorously indecent
    Lewd *(adjective)*
    Obscene *(adjective)*
    Indecent *(adjective)*
    Coarse *(adjective)*

Beacon *(noun)*–A fire or light set up in a high or prominent position as a warning, signal or celebration
    Flare *(noun)*
    Bonfire *(noun)*
    Beam *(noun)*
    Signal fire *(noun)*

Bedlam *(noun)*–A scene of uproar and confusion
    Pandemonium *(noun)*
    Commotion *(noun)*
    Mayhem *(noun)*
    Unrest *(noun)*

Behemoth *(noun)*–Giant
    Beast *(noun)*
    Monster *(noun)*
    Huge *(noun)*
    Mammoth *(noun)*

Beholden *(adjective)*–Indebted
    Grateful *(adjective)*
    Owing *(adjective)*
    Bound *(adjective)*
    Obligated *(adjective)*

Behoove *(verb)* –Be necessary, proper
    Befit *(verb)*
    Beseem *(verb)*
    Suit *(verb)*
    Ask *(verb)*

Belittle *(verb)* –Detract
    Criticize *(verb)*
    Derogate *(verb)*
    Smear *(verb)*
    Deride *(verb)*

Belligerent *(adjective)*–Nasty, agumentative
    Aggressive *(adjective)*
    Quarrelsome *(adjective)*
    Bellicose *(adjective)*
    Hostile *(adjective)*

Bemoan *(verb)* –Express sorrow
    Deplore *(verb)*
    Bewail *(verb)*
    Mourn *(verb)*
    Rue *(verb)*

Bemused *(adjective)*–Absent minded
    Distracted *(adjective)*
    Abstracted *(adjective)*

Preoccupied *(adjective)*
Dreamy *(adjective)*

Benign *(adjective)*–Kindly
Benevolent *(adjective)*
Generous (*adjective*)
Kind (*adjective*)
Favourable *(adjective)*

Benevolent *(adjective)*–Charitable, kind
Caring (*adjective*)
Humane *(adjective)*
Generous (*adjective*)
Humanitarian *(adjective)*

Berate (*verb*) –Criticize hatefully
Reproach *(verb)*
Reprove *(verb)*
Castigate *(verb)*
Scorch *(verb)*

Beseech *(verb)* –Beg
Implore *(verb)*
Appeal *(verb)*
Ask *(verb)*
Invoke *(verb)*

Besmirch *(verb)* –Taint
Blacken (*verb*)
Slander (*verb*)
Stain (*verb*)
Defile *(verb)*

Bestow *(verb)* –Give, allot
Lavish *(verb)*
Favour *(verb)*
Confer *(verb)*
Donate *(verb)*

Bias *(noun)*–Belief in one way; partiality
Penchant *(noun)*
Tilt *(noun)*
Bigotry *(noun)*
Leaning *(noun)*

Bicker (*verb*) –Nastily argue
Disagree *(verb)*
Altercate (*verb*)
Fight (*verb*)
Tiff *(verb)*

Bifurcate *(verb)* –Divide into two branches
Divide (*verb*)
Bisect (*verb*)
Ramify (*verb*)
Branch *(verb)*

Bilateral *(adjective)*–Having two sides
Mutual *(adjective)*
Respective *(adjective)*
Reciprocal *(adjective)*
Two-sided *(adjective)*

Billowing *(verb)* –Surge
Undulate *(verb)*
Bulge (*verb*)
Roll (*verb*)
Bloat *(verb)*

Binge *(noun)*–Spree
Orgy (*noun*)
Affair (*noun*)
Bender (*noun*)
Drunk *(noun)*

Bland *(adjective)*–Tasteless; undistinctive
Banal (*adjective*)
Boring (*adjective*)
Dull (*adjective*)
Insipid (*adjective*)

Blare (*verb*) –Make loud noise
Bark *(verb)*
Roar (*verb*)
Trumpet (*verb*)
Clang *(verb)*

Blasphemy *(noun)*–Irreverance
  Heresy *(noun)*
  Scoffing *(noun)*
  Abuse *(noun)*
  Swearing *(noun)*

Bleak *(adjective)*–Barren
  Cold *(adjective)*
  Austere *(adjective)*
  Chilly *(adjective)*
  Stripped *(adjective)*

Blatant *(adjective)*–Obvious; brazen
  Outright *(adjective)*
  Loud *(adjective)*
  Barefaced *(adjective)*
  Pronounced *(adjective)*

Belch *(verb)* –Emit wind noisily from the stomach through the mouth
  Rift *(noun)*
  Burp *(verb)*
  Bring up wind *(verb)*
  Gurk *(verb)*

Beleaguer *(verb)* –Lay siege to
  Besieged *(verb)*
  Blockaded *(verb)*
  Under attack *(verb)*
  Hemmed in *(verb)*

Bereft *(adjective)*–Deprived of or lacking something
  Robbed of *(adjective)*
  Stripped of *(adjective)*
  Lacking *(adjective)*
  Deficient in *(adjective)*

Bevy *(noun)*–A large group of people or things of a particular kind
  Gang *(noun)*

  Party *(noun)*
  Crowd *(noun)*
  Pack *(noun)*

Bigot *(noun)*–A person who is intolerant of any differing creed, belief or opinion
  Dogmatist *(noun)*
  Partisan *(noun)*
  Sectarian *(noun)*
  Prejudiced person *(noun)*

Billowing *(verb)* –Fill with air and swell outwards
  Puff up *(verb)*
  Bulge out *(verb)*
  Belly out *(verb)*
  Balloon out *(verb)*

Blanched *(verb)* –Flinch or grow pale from shock, fear or a similar reaction
  Shrink *(verb)*
  Recoil *(verb)*
  Wince *(verb)*
  Start *(verb)*

Blighted *(verb)* –Spoil, harm or destroy
  Ruin *(verb)*
  Wreck *(verb)*
  Mar *(verb)*
  Devastate *(verb)*

Blinder *(noun)*–Blinker's on a horse's bridle
  Hood *(noun)*
  Shade *(noun)*
  Blindfold *(noun)*
  Bluff *(noun)*

Blazon *(verb)* –Display prominently or vividly
- Exhibit *(verb)*
- Flaunt *(verb)*
- Parade *(verb)*
- Reveal *(verb)*

Blithesome *(adjective)*–Carefree and happy and lighthearted
- Cheerful *(adjective)*
- Jovial *(adjective)*
- Merry *(adjective)*
- Mirthful *(adjective)*

Braggadocio *(noun)*–Boastful or arrogant behaviour
- Boaster *(noun)*
- Bragger *(noun)*
- Show-off *(noun)*
- Windbag *(noun)*

Bridle *(noun)*–The headgear used to control a horse
- Control *(noun)*
- Curb *(noun)*
- Halter *(noun)*
- Rein *(noun)*

Brigand *(noun)*–A member of a gang that ambushes and robs people in forests and mountains
- Bandit *(noun)*
- Desperado *(noun)*
- Robber *(noun)*
- Highwayman *(noun)*

Brindle *(noun)*–A brownish colour of animal fur, with streaks of other colour
- Motley *(adjective)*
- Checkered *(adjective)*
- Spotted *(adjective)*
- Speckled *(adjective)*

Brio *(noun)*–Vigour or vivacity of style or performance
- Gusto *(noun)*
- Verve *(noun)*
- Animation *(noun)*
- Zest *(noun)*

Brook *(noun)*–A small stream
- Small river *(noun)*
- Brooklet *(noun)*
- Runlet *(noun)*
- Creek *(noun)*

Brusque *(adjective)*–Abrupt or offhand in speech or manner
- Curt *(adjective)*
- Blunt *(adjective)*
- Sharp *(adjective)*
- Terse *(adjective)*

Buck *(verb)* –Oppose or resist
- Contradict *(verb)*
- Defy *(verb)*
- Fight against *(verb)*
- Go against *(verb)*

Buffoon *(noun)*–A ridiculous but amusing person
- Clown *(noun)*
- Fool *(noun)*
- Jester *(noun)*
- Joker *(noun)*

Bungle *(verb)* –Carry out a task clumsily or incompetently
- Mishandle *(verb)*
- Mismanage *(verb)*
- Botch *(verb)*
- Spoil *(verb)*

Burgeon *(verb)* –Begin to grow or increase rapidly
- Flourish *(verb)*
- Expand *(verb)*
- Swell *(verb)*
- Proliferate *(verb)*

Burly *(adjective)*–A large and strong, heavily-built person
- Strapping *(adjective)*
- Brawny *(adjective)*
- Muscular *(adjective)*
- Stocky *(adjective)*

Button *(noun)*–A small device on an electrical equipment which is pressed to operate it
- Knob *(noun)*
- Switch *(noun)*
- Control *(noun)*
- Lever *(noun)*

C

Caitiff *(noun)*–A contemptible or cowardly person
  Dastard *(noun)*
  Louse *(noun)*
  Rat *(noun)*
  Scoundrel *(noun)*

Carnal *(adjective)*–Relating to physical, especially sexual, needs and activities
  Sensual *(adjective)*
  Erotic *(adjective)*
  Lascivious *(adjective)*
  Lewd *(adjective)*

Cardinal *(adjective)*–Of the greatest importance; fundamental
  Main *(adjective)*
  Chief *(adjective)*
  Primary *(adjective)*
  Paramount *(adjective)*

Caveat *(noun)*–A warning or proviso of specific conditions or limitations
  Warning *(adjective)*
  Caution *(noun)*
  Admonition *(noun)*
  Red flag *(noun)*

Cabal *(noun)*–A secret political clique or faction
  Group *(noun)*
  Party *(noun)*
  Band *(noun)*
  Coterie *(noun)*

Cachet *(noun)*–The state of being respected or admired
  Prestige *(noun)*
  Distinction *(noun)*
  Status *(noun)*
  Eminence *(noun)*

Cacophonous *(adjective)*–Harsh sounding
  Discordant *(adjective)*
  Disharmonic *(adjective)*
  Noisy *(adjective)*
  Clinking *(adjective)*

Calamity *(noun)*–Disaster; tragedy
  Adversity *(noun)*
  Scourge *(noun)*
  Misadventure *(noun)*
  Mishap *(noun)*

Callow *(adjective)*–Immature
  Inexperienced *(adjective)*
  Jellybean *(adjective)*
  Naive *(adjective)*
  Infant *(adjective)*

Calm *(adjective)*–Peaceful, quiet
Mild *(adjective)*
  Placid *(adjective)*
  Serene *(adjective)*
  Tranquil *(adjective)*

Calumny *(noun)*–The making of false statements about someone in

order to damage their reputation
Slander *(noun)*
Defamation *(noun)*
Character assassination *(noun)*
Libel *(noun)*

Cantankerous *(adjective)*–Bad-tempered, argumentative and unco-operative
Irascible *(adjective)*
Irritable *(adjective)*
Grumpy *(adjective)*
Grouchy *(adjective)*

Canonry *(noun)*–The office of a canon
Cardinalate *(noun)*
Pastorate *(noun)*
Deaconry *(noun)*
Diaconate *(noun)*

Carousal *(noun)*–A merry drinking party
Binge *(noun)*
Spree *(noun)*
Revel *(noun)*
Bender *(noun)*

Careen *(verb)* –Move swiftly and in an uncontrolled way
Lurch *(verb)*
Pitch *(verb)*
Sway *(verb)*
Tilt *(verb)*

Catacomb *(noun)*–An underground cemetery with recesses for tombs
Sepulchre *(noun)*
Crypt *(noun)*
Vault *(noun)*
Mausoleum *(noun)*

Catchword *(noun)*–A popular word or phrase encapsulating a par-ticular concept
Slogan *(noun)*
mantra *(noun)*
Maxim *(noun)*
Motto *(noun)*

Catechism *(noun)*–A summary of the principles of the Christian religion in the form of questions and answers
Belief *(noun)*
Principles *(noun)*
Tenet *(noun)*
Doctrine *(noun)*

Castigate *(verb)* –Criticize severely
Berate *(verb)*
Rebuke *(verb)*
Drub *(verb)*
Reprimand *(verb)*

Caustic *(adjective)*–Burning corrosive
Abrasive *(adjective)*
Acerbic *(adjective)*
Biting *(adjective)*
Pungent *(adjective)*

Cease *(verb)* –Stop, conclude
Discontinue *(verb)*
Halt *(verb)*
Refrain *(verb)*
Finish *(verb)*

Cede *(verb)* –Abandon, surrender
Capitulate *(verb)*
Drop *(verb)*
Concede *(verb)*
Grant *(verb)*

Cheap *(adjective)*–Inexpensive
Competitive *(adjective)*
Economical *(adjective)*
Reasonable *(adjective)*
bargain *(noun)*

Cheerful *(adjective)*–Happy
  Animated *(adjective)*
  Cheery *(adjective)*
  Lively *(adjective)*
  Merry *(adjective)*

Clear *(adjective)*–Cloudless, bright
  Sunny *(adjective)*
  Fine *(adjective)*
  Pleasant *(adjective)*
  Halcyon *(adjective)*

Clumsy *(adjective)*–Not agile, awkward
  Inept *(adjective)*
  Ungainly *(adjective)*
  gawky *(adjective)*
  Graceless *(adjective)*

Conceal *(verb)* –Hide, disguise
  Cloak *(verb)*
  Cover *(verb)*
  Mask *(verb)*
  Enshroud *(verb)*

Crooked *(adjective)*–Bent, angled
  Curved *(adjective)*
  Gnarled *(adjective)*
  Twisted *(adjective)*
  Deformed *(adjective)*

Compulsory *(adjective)*–Binding
  Forced *(adjective)*
  Imperative *(adjective)*
  mandatory *(adjective)*
  Obligatory *(adjective)*

Candid *(adjective)*–Honest
  Blunt *(adjective)*
  Forthright *(adjective)*
  Bluff *(adjective)*
  Equal *(adjective)*

Capable *(adjective)*–Able to perform
  Accomplished *(adjective)*
  Adept *(adjective)*
  Competent *(adjective)*
  Efficient *(adjective)*

Captive *(adjective)*–Physically held by force
  Imprisoned *(adjective)*
  Bound *(adjective)*
  Confined *(adjective)*
  Enslaved *(adjective)*

Capitulate *(verb)* –Give in
  Relent *(verb)*
  Bow *(verb)*
  Concede *(verb)*
  Defer *(verb)*

Capricious *(adjective)*–Given to sudden behaviour change
  Arbitrary *(adjective)*
  Unstable *(adjective)*
  Mutable *(adjective)*
  Fickle *(adjective)*

Chagrin *(noun)*–Displeasure
  Blow *(noun)*
  Crushing *(noun)*
  Dismay *(noun)*
  Irritation *(noun)*

Charisma *(noun)*–Great personal charm
  Glamour *(noun)*
  Dazzle *(noun)*
  Allure *(noun)*
  Magnetism *(noun)*

Chastise *(verb)* –Scold, discipline
  Flog *(verb)*
  Lash *(verb)*
  Punish *(verb)*
  Baste *(verb)*

Chronic *(adjective)*–Incessant, never-ending
  Constant *(adjective)*

Incurable *(adjective)*
Habitual *(adjective)*
Enduring *(adjective)*

Circumspect *(adjective)*–Cautious, discreet
Prudent (*adjective*)
Vigilant (*adjective*)
Cagey (*adjective*)
Safe *(adjective)*

Clandestine (*adjective*)–Secret, sly
Covert (*adjective*)
Foxy (*adjective*)
Sneaky (*adjective*)
Hidden *(adjective)*

Clemency (*noun*)–Forgiveness
Compassion (*noun*)
Forbearance (*noun*)
Mercy (*noun*)
Charity *(noun)*

Clique (*noun*)–Group of friends
Clan (*noun*)
Mafia (*noun*)
Bunch (*noun*)
Circle *(noun)*

Coercion (*noun*)–Compulsion, pressure
Duress (*noun*)
Constraint (*noun*)
Threat (*noun*)
Intimidation *(noun)*

Caucus *(noun)*–A group of people with shared concerns within a political party or larger organization
Meeting *(noun)*
Assembly *(noun)*
Convention *(noun)*
Congregation *(noun)*

Cauldron *(noun)*–A large metal plot with a lid and handle, used for cooking over an open fire
Vessel *(noun)*
Utensil *(noun)*
Beaker *(noun)*
Carafe *(noun)*

Causeway *(noun)*–A raised road or track across low or wet ground
Hill *(noun)*
Bank *(noun)*
Breakwater *(noun)*
Mound *(noun)*

Cavil *(verb)* –Make petty or unnecessary objections
Complain *(verb)*
Carp *(verb)*
Grumble *(verb)*
Whine *(verb)*

Certitude *(noun)*–Absolute certainty or conviction that something is the case
Confidence *(noun)*
Assurance *(noun)*
Conviction *(noun)*
Reliable *(adjective)*

Chary *(adjective)*–Cautiously or suspiciously reluctant to do something
Circumspect *(adjective)*
Heedful *(adjective)*
Guarded *(adjective)*
Mindful *(adjective)*

Chateau *(noun)*–A large French country house or castle, often giving its name to wine made in its neighbourhood
Estate *(noun)*
manor *(noun)*
Mansion *(noun)*
Villa *(noun)*

Chatoyant *(adjective)*–A band of bright luster in a gem caused by reflection from inclusions in the stone
    Gleaming *(adjective)*
    Glistening *(adjective)*
    Lustrous *(adjective)*
    Burnished *(adjective)*

Chagrin *(noun)*–Annoyance or distress at having failed or being humiliated
    Anger *(noun)*
    Rage *(noun)*
    Displeasure *(noun)*
    Fury *(noun)*

Chafe *(verb)* –Make or become sore by rubbing against something
    Scrape *(verb)*
    Scratch *(verb)*
    Rasp *(verb)*
    Graze *(verb)*

Charlatan *(noun)*–A person falsely claiming to have a special knowledge or skill
    Quack *(noun)*
    Fraud *(noun)*
    Humbug *(noun)*
    Imposter *(noun)*

Cherub *(noun)*–A winged angelic being described in biblical tradition as attending on God
    Angel *(noun)*
    Seraph *(noun)*
    Sprite *(noun)*
    Archangel *(noun)*

Christened *(verb)* –Give a baby a Christian name at baptism as a sign of admission to a Christian Church
    Baptize *(verb)*

    Bless *(verb)*
    Designate *(verb)*
    Immerse *(verb)*

Chimerical *(adjective)*–Being or relating to or like a chimera
    Utopian *(adjective)*
    Mythical *(adjective)*
    Imaginary *(adjective)*
    Fantastic *(adjective)*

Churlish *(adjective)*–Rude in a mean-spirited and churlish way
    Discourteous *(adjective)*
    Impolite *(adjective)*
    Uncivil *(adjective)*
    Rude *(adjective)*

Clandestine *(adjective)*–Kept secret or done secretively
    Covert *(adjective)*
    Furtive *(adjective)*
    Stealthy *(adjective)*
    Concealed *(adjective)*

Clime *(noun)*–A region considered with reference to its climate
    Conditions *(noun)*
    Characteristic weather *(noun)*
    Atmospheric conditions *(noun)*
    Meteorologic conditions *(noun)*

Clobber *(verb)* –Hit someone hard
    Thrash *(verb)*
    Wallop *(verb)*
    Slug *(verb)*
    Smash *(verb)*

Codicil *(noun)*–An addition or supplement that explains, modifies, or revokes a will
    Addendum *(noun)*
    Postscript *(noun)*
    Rider *(noun)*
    Appendix *(noun)*

Coffer *(noun)*–A strongbox or chest for holding valuables
- Casket *(noun)*
- Trunk *(noun)*
- Safe *(noun)*
- Repository *(noun)*

Comity *(noun)*–An association of nations for their mutual benefit
- Concord *(noun)*
- Goodwill *(noun)*
- Harmony *(noun)*
- Cordiality *(noun)*

Commensurate *(adjective)*–Corresponding in size or degree
- Equivalent *(adjective)*
- Comparable *(adjective)*
- Equal *(adjective)*
- Proportionate *(adjective)*

Compunction *(noun)*–A feeling of guilt or moral scruple that prevents or follows the doing of something bad
- Misgivings *(noun)*
- Qualms *(noun)*
- Unease *(noun)*
- Reservations *(noun)*

Conation *(noun)*–The mental faculty of purpose, desire or will to perform an action
- Intention
- Plan *(noun)*
- Volition *(noun)*
- Will *(noun)*

Conceit *(noun)*–Excessive pride in oneself
- Vanity *(noun)*
- Narcissism *(noun)*
- Egotism *(noun)*
- Egomania *(noun)*

Concomitant *(noun)*–A phenomenon that naturally accompanies or follows something
- Associated *(verb)*
- Collateral *(adjective)*
- Related *(adjective)*
- Linked *(adjective)*

Conduit *(noun)*–A channel for conveying water or other fluid
- Duct *(noun)*
- Pipe *(noun)*
- Tube *(noun)*
- Chute *(noun)*

Condole *(verb)* –Express sympathy for someone
- Soothe *(verb)*
- Commiserate *(verb)*
- Console *(verb)*
- Comfort *(verb)*

Connotative *(adjective)*–Having the power of implying or suggesting something in addition to what is explicit
- Hinting *(verb)*
- Implying *(verb)*
- Referring *(verb)*
- Suggesting *(verb)*

Construe *(verb)* –Interpret a word or action in a particular way
- Analyse *(verb)*
- Decode *(verb)*
- Elucidate *(verb)*
- Explain *(verb)*

Consort *(noun)*–A wife, husband or companion, in particular the spouse of a reigning monarch
- Partner *(noun)*
- Companion *(noun)*

Mate *(noun)*
Spouse *(noun)*

Contrivance *(noun)*–The use of skill to create or bring about something
  Scheme *(noun)*
  Tactic *(noun)*
  Plan *(noun)*
  Ploy *(noun)*

Convalesce *(verb)* –Recover one's health and strength over a period of time after an illness or medical treatment
  Recover *(verb)*
  Recuperate *(verb)*
  Revive *(verb)*
  Restore *(verb)*

Conflux *(noun)*–The junction of two rivers, especially rivers of approximately equal width
  Convergence *(noun)*
  Confluence *(noun)*
  Junction *(noun)*
  Watersmeet *(noun)*

Concourse *(noun)*–A large open area inside or in front of a public building
  Entrance *(noun)*
  Foyer *(noun)*
  Lobby *(noun)*
  Hall *(noun)*

Contingency *(noun)*–A future event or circumstance which is possible but cannot be predicted with certainty
  Eventuality *(noun)*
  Occurrence *(noun)*
  Possibility *(noun)*
  Happening *(noun)*

Countervail *(verb)* –Offset the effect of something by countering it with something of equal force
  Counteract *(verb)*
  Neutralize *(verb)*
  Nullify *(verb)*
  Counterbalance *(verb)*

Countenance *(noun)*–A person's face or facial expression
  Physiognomy *(noun)*
  Profile *(noun)*
  Visage *(noun)*
  Demeanour *(noun)*

Counterpoise *(noun)*–A factor or force that balances or neutralizes another
  Balance *(noun)*
  Equalization *(noun)*
  Counteraction *(noun)*
  Offset *(noun)*

Countermand *(verb)* –Revoke or cancel an order
  Rescind *(verb)*
  Repeal *(verb)*
  Retract *(verb)*
  Override *(verb)*

Cohorts *(noun)*–A group of people with a shared characteristic
  Unit *(noun)*
  Outfit *(noun)*
  Force *(noun)*
  Crew *(noun)*

Covetousness *(noun)*–An envious eagerness to possess something
  Avariciousness *(noun)*
  Cupidity *(noun)*
  Greed *(noun)*
  Jealousy *(noun)*

Credenda *(noun)*–Any of the sections into which a creed or other statement of doctrine is divided
    Axiom *(noun)*
    Dogma *(noun)*
    Tenet *(noun)*
    Canon *(noun)*

Cupola *(noun)*–A rounded dome forming or adorning a roof or ceiling
    Dome *(noun)*
    Belfry *(noun)*
    Bulge *(noun)*
    Bubble *(noun)*

Curtail *(verb)* –Reduce in extent or quantity
    Decrease *(verb)*
    Lessen *(verb)*
    Diminish *(verb)*
    Retrench *(verb)*

Cull *(verb)* –Select from a large quantity
    Choose *(verb)*
    Pick *(verb)*
    Glean *(verb)*
    Take *(verb)*

Curio *(noun)*–A rare, unusual or intriguing object
    Trinket *(noun)*
    Ornament *(noun)*
    Bauble *(noun)*
    Knick knack *(noun)*

D

Daintily *(adverb)* –In a refined manner
   Elegantly *(adverb)*
   Exquisitely *(adverb)*
   Finely *(adverb)*
   Delicately *(adverb)*

Dangerous *(adjective)*–Hazardous, troubling
   Alarming *(adjective)*
   Bad *(adjective)*
   Critical *(adjective)*
   Unsafe *(adjective)*

Decline *(noun)*–Lessening
   Deterioration *(noun)*
   Downturn *(noun)*
   Failure *(noun)*
   Slump *(noun)*

Definite *(adjective)*–Exact, clear
   Definitive *(adjective)*
   Obvious *(adjective)*
   Positive *(adjective)*
   Precise *(adjective)*

Despair *(noun)*–Depression, hopelessness
   Anguish *(noun)*
   Despondency *(noun)*
   Gloom *(noun)*
   Misery *(noun)*

Dreary *(adjective)*–Gloomy, lifeless
   Bleak *(adjective)*
   Boring *(adjective)*

Dismal *(adjective)*
   Tedious *(adjective)*

Dull *(adjective)*–Unintelligent
   Dumb *(adjective)*
   Simple *(adjective)*
   Slow *(adjective)*
   Addled *(adjective)*

Discourage *(verb)* –Dishearten, dispirit
   Dampen *(verb)*
   Demoralize *(verb)*
   Intimidate *(verb)*
   Unnerve *(verb)*

Dim *(adjective)*–Darkish
   Dark *(adjective)*
   Dingy *(adjective)*
   Gloomy *(adjective)*
   Shadowy *(adjective)*

Dark *(adjective)*–Lack of light
   Cloudy *(adjective)*
   darkened *(adjective)*
   Somber *(adjective)*
   Dusky *(adjective)*

Demand *(noun)*–Question, request
   Appeal *(noun)*
   Insistence *(noun)*
   Need *(noun)*
   Requirement *(noun)*

Daub *(noun)*–A patch or smear of a thick or sticky substance
   Splash *(noun)*

Daft → Delirium

Stain *(noun)*
Coat *(noun)*
Spatter *(noun)*

Daft *(adjective)*–Silly; foolish
Absurd *(adjective)*
Ridiculous *(adjective)*
Ludicrous *(adjective)*
Stupid *(adjective)*

Dapple *(verb)* –Mark with spots or rounded patches
Dot *(noun)*
Fleck *(noun)*
Streak *(noun)*
Speck *(noun)*

Deaconry *(noun)*–The office or position of a deacon or minister of the church
Priesthood *(noun)*
Pastorate *(noun)*
Canonry *(noun)*
Diaconate *(noun)*

Debark *(verb)* –Leave a ship or aircraft
Arrive *(verb)*
Disembark *(verb)*
Go ashore *(verb)*

Debilitating *(adjective)*–A disease or condition that makes one weak and infirm
Devitalize *(verb)*
Enfeeble *(verb)*
Weaken *(verb)*
Unstrengthen *(verb)*

Denizen *(noun)*–A person, animal or plant that lives or is found in a particular place
Inhabitant *(noun)*
Resident *(noun)*

Native *(noun)*
Local *(noun)*

Descry *(verb)* –Catch sight of
Behold *(verb)*
Detect *(verb)*
Discern *(verb)*
Perceive *(verb)*

Depredation *(verb)* –An act of attacking or plundering
Looting *(verb)*
Pillaging *(verb)*
Robbing *(verb)*
Ravaging *(verb)*

Decrepit *(adjective)*–Worn out or ruined because of age or neglect
Dilapidated *(adjective)*
Ramshackle *(adjective)*
Derelict *(adjective)*
Ruined *(adjective)*

Decry *(verb)* –Publicly denounce
Condemn *(verb)*
Criticize *(verb)*
Censure *(verb)*
Deplore *(verb)*

Denigration *(noun)*–A belitting comment
Defamation *(noun)*
Aspersion *(noun)*
Slander *(noun)*
Disparagement *(noun)*

Delirium *(noun)*–An acutely disturbed state of mind characterized by restlessness, illusions and incoherence occurring in intoxication, fever and other disorders
Derangement *(noun)*
Dementia *(noun)*
Insanity *(noun)*
Dementedness *(noun)*

Deposed *(verb)* –Remove from office suddenly and forcefully
- Overthrow *(verb)*
- Overturn *(verb)*
- Displace *(verb)*
- Dethrone *(verb)*

Devolution *(noun)*–The transfer or delegation of power to a lower level
- Surrender *(noun)*
- Relinquishment *(noun)*
- Downgrade *(noun)*
- Regress *(noun)*

Diatribe *(noun)*–A forceful and bitter verbal attack against someone or something
- Tirade *(noun)*
- Harangue *(noun)*
- Reproof *(noun)*
- Reprimand *(noun)*

Diabolical *(adjective)*–Characteristic of the devil; disgracefully bad or unpleasant
- Devilish *(adjective)*
- Fiendish *(adjective)*
- Satanic *(adjective)*
- Demonic *(adjective)*

Dominion *(noun)*–the territory of a sovereign or government
- Protectorate *(noun)*
- Province *(noun)*
- Outpost *(noun)*
- Colony *(noun)*

Dour *(adjective)*–relentlessly severe, stern or gloomy in manner or appearance
- Forbidding *(Adjective)*
- Morose *(adjective)*
- Sullen *(adjective)*
- Stony *(adjective)*

E

Ebb *(noun)*–the movement of the tide out to sea
    Receding *(verb)*
    Subsiding *(verb)*
    Retreating *(verb)*
    Abating *(verb)*

Ecclesiastic *(noun)*–a priest or clergyman
    Cleric *(noun)*
    Minister *(noun)*
    Preacher *(noun)*
    Chaplain *(noun)*

Edacity *(noun)*–excessive desire to eat
    Rapaciousness *(noun)*
    Ravenousness *(noun)*
    Gluttonousness *(noun)*
    Insatiability *(noun)*

Edifice *(noun)*–a large imposing building
    Structure *(noun)*
    Pile *(noun)*
    Structure *(noun)*
    Complex *(noun)*

Elegant *(adjective)*–beautiful, tasteful
    Chic *(adjective)*
    Exquisite *(adjective)*
    Graceful *(adjective)*
    Refined *(adjective)*

Elementary *(adjective)*–simple, basic
    Elemental *(adjective)*
    Fundamental *(adjective)*
    Rudimentary *(adjective)*
    Straightforward *(adjective)*

Encourage *(verb)* –stimulate spiritually
    Boost *(verb)*
    Inspire *(verb)*
    Spur *(verb)*
    Push *(verb)*

Enemy *(noun)*–someone hated or competed against
    Adversary *(noun)*
    Antagonist *(noun)*
    Foe *(noun)*
    Opponent *(noun)*

Entrance *(noun)*–a way into a place
    Access *(noun)*
    Door *(noun)*
    Entry *(noun)*
    Gate *(noun)*

Equal *(adjective)*–alike
    Balanced *(adjective)*
    Comparable *(adjective)*
    Equivalent *(adjective)*
    Proportional *(adjective)*

Excited *(adjective)*–Inspired, upset
    Delighted *(adjective)*
    Enthusiastic *(adjective)*
    Passionate *(adjective)*
    Charged *(adjective)*

Expand *(verb)* –Extend, augment
    Broaden *(verb)*
    Enlarge *(verb)*
    Increase *(verb)*
    Spread *(verb)*

Export *(verb)* –Sell or trade abroad
    Ship *(verb)*
    Transport *(verb)*
    Dump *(verb)*
    Freight *(verb)*

Exterior *(adjective)*–Outside
    External *(adjective)*
    Outdoor *(adjective)*
    Outer *(adjective)*
    Peripheral surface *(adjective)*

Emblematic *(adjective)*–Serving as a symbol of a particular quality or concept
    Symbolic *(adjective)*
    Representative *(adjective)*
    Indicative *(adjective)*
    Symptomatic *(adjective)*

Errand *(noun)*–A short journey undertaken in order to deliver or collect something, especially on someone else's behalf
    Task *(noun)*
    Chore *(noun)*
    Job *(noun)*
    Assignment *(noun)*

Eschew *(verb)* –Deliberately avoid using; abstain from
    Forgo *(verb)*

    Shun *(verb)*
    Renounce *(verb)*
    Relinquish *(verb)*

Espouse *(verb)* –Adopt or support a cause, belief or way of life
    Embrace *(verb)*
    Accept *(verb)*
    Welcome *(verb)*
    Endorse *(verb)*

Epicure *(noun)*–A person who takes particular pleasure in fine food and drink
    Gourmet *(noun)*
    Gastronome *(noun)*
    Gourmand *(noun)*
    Connoisseur *(noun)*

Encumbrance *(noun)*–An impediment or burden
    Hindrance *(noun)*
    Obstruction *(noun)*
    Obstacle *(noun)*
    Constraint *(noun)*

Endowment *(noun)*–The action of endowing something or someone
    Funding *(noun)*
    Financing *(noun)*
    Subsidizing *(noun)*
    Donation *(noun)*

Envisage *(verb)* –Contemplate or conceive of as a possibility or a desirable future event
    Foresee *(verb)*
    Predict *(verb)*
    Forecast *(verb)*
    Anticipate *(verb)*

Enunciation *(noun)*–The articulation of speech regarded from the point of view of its intelligibility to

the audience
Elocution *(noun)*
Pronunciation *(noun)*
Fluency *(noun)*
Voicing *(noun)*

Esoteric *(adjective)*–Intended for or likely to be understood by only a small number of people with a specialized knowledge or interest
Abstruse *(adjective)*
Obscure *(adjective)*
Rarefied *(adjective)*
Enigmatic *(adjective)*

Evince *(verb)* –Reveal the presence of a quality or feeling
Manifest *(verb)*
Display *(verb)*
Exhibit *(verb)*
Demonstrate *(verb)*

Exacting *(adjective)*–Making great demands on one's skill, attention and other resources
Demanding *(adjective)*
Challenging *(adjective)*
Taxing *(adjective)*
Gruelling *(adjective)*

Exacerbate *(verb)* –Make a problem or bad situation worse
Aggravate *(verb)*
Worsen *(verb)*
Inflame *(verb)*
Compound *(verb)*

Excoriate *(verb)* –Damage or remove part of the surface
Abrade *(verb)*
Scrape *(verb)*
Scratch *(verb)*
Chafe *(verb)*

Exegesis *(noun)*–Critical explanation or interpretation of a text, especially of scripture
Exposition *(noun)*
Elucidation *(noun)*
Clarification *(noun)*
Explanation *(noun)*

Exhort *(verb)* –Strongly encourage or urge someone to do something
Persuade *(verb)*
Pressurize *(verb)*
Push *(verb)*
Spur *(verb)*

Expunge *(verb)* –Obliterate or remove completely
Erase *(verb)*
Delete *(verb)*
Wipe out *(verb)*
Efface *(verb)*

Expurgate *(verb)* –Remove matter thought to be objectionable or unsuitable
Censor *(verb)*
Redact *(verb)*
Cut *(verb)*
Edit *(verb)*

Extol *(verb)* –Praise enthusiastically
Eulogize *(verb)*
Rhapsodize *(verb)*
Rave *(verb)*
Gush *(verb)*

Extemporary *(adjective)*–Spoken or done without preparation
Impromptu *(adjective)*
Spontaneous *(adjective)*
Unscripted *(adjective)*
Ad lib *(adjective)*

F

Fade *(verb)* –Lose colour
    Disappear *(verb)*
    Evaporate *(verb)*
    Vanish *(verb)*
    Neutralize *(verb)*

Famished *(adjective)*–Starving
    Empty *(adjective)*
    Hollow *(adjective)*
    Hungering *(adjective)*
    Ravening *(adjective)*

Fat *(adjective)*–Overweight
    Big *(adjective)*
    Bulky *(adjective)*
    Hefty *(adjective)*
    large *(adjective)*

Feeble *(adjective)*–Not strong, ineffective
    Ailing *(adjective)*
    Weak *(adjective)*
    Fragile *(adjective)*
    Frail *(adjective)*

Float *(verb)* –Lie on the surface
    Drift *(verb)*
    Glide *(verb)*
    Slide *(verb)*
    Swim *(verb)*

Foolish *(adjective)*–Nonsensical, idiotic
    Absurd *(adjective)*
    Crazy *(adjective)*
    Insane *(adjective)*
    Silly *(adjective)*

Forget *(verb)* –Not be able to remember
    Obliterate *(verb)*
    Dismiss from mind *(verb)*
    Draw a blank *(verb)*
    Let slip from memory *(verb)*

Fresh *(adjective)*–New, just produced
    Crisp *(adjective)*
    Green *(adjective)*
    Natural *(adjective)*
    Raw *(adjective)*

Frequent *(adjective)*–Common, repeated
    Commonplace *(adjective)*
    Incessant *(adjective)*
    Periodic *(adjective)*
    Usual *(adjective)*

Fortunate *(adjective)*–Having good luck
    Fortuitous *(adjective)*
    Lucky *(adjective)*
    Well-off *(adjective)*
    Advantageous *(adjective)*

Fecund *(adjective)*–Producing or capable of producing an abundance of offspring or new growth; highly fertile
    Prolific *(adjective)*
    Propagating *(adjective)*
    Fruitful *(adjective)*

Proliferant *(adjective)*

Festoon *(verb)* –Adorn with chains, garlands or other decorations
Decorate *(verb)*
Dress up *(verb)*
Deck out *(verb)*
Bedeck *(verb)*

Fetid *(adjective)*–Smelling extremely unpleasant
Smelly *(adjective)*
Malodorous *(adjective)*
Rank *(adjective)*
Foul *(adjective)*

Fiery *(adjective)*–Consisting of fire or burning strongly and brightly
Blazing *(adjective)*
Flaming *(adjective)*
Raging *(adjective)*
Ablaze *(adjective)*

Flintlock *(noun)*–An old-fashioned type of gun fired by a spark from a flint
Handgun *(noun)*
Musket *(noun)*
Pistol *(noun)*
Revolver *(noun)*

Flummox *(verb)* –Perplex someone greatly
Bewilder *(verb)*
Baffle *(verb)*
Mystify *(verb)*
Disconcert *(verb)*

Foray *(noun)*–A sudden attack or incursion into enemy territory, especially to obtain something

Raid *(noun)*
Attack *(noun)*
Assault *(noun)*
Swoop *(noun)*

Fount *(noun)*–A source of a desirable quality or commodity
Fountain *(noun)*
Wellspring *(noun)*
Spring *(noun)*
Well *(noun)*

Fractious *(adjective)*–Irritable and quarrelsome
Grumpy *(adjective)*
Grouchy *(adjective)*
Peevish *(adjective)*
Petty *(adjective)*

Funambulist *(noun)*–A tightrope walker
Gymnast *(noun)*
Aerialist *(noun)*
Stunt person *(noun)*
Contortionist *(noun)*

Fuliginous *(adjective)*–Sooty; dusky
Smoky *(adjective)*
Vague *(adjective)*
Clouded *(adjective)*
Murky *(adjective)*

Furtive *(adjective)*–Attempting to avoid notice or attention
Secretive *(adjective)*
Surreptitious *(adjective)*
Sneaky *(adjective)*

G

Wily *(adjective)*

Garotte *(verb)* –Kill someone by strangulation, especially with a length of wire or cord
Behead *(verb)*
Decapitate *(verb)*
Lynch *(verb)*
Asphyxiate *(verb)*

Gasp *(noun)*–A convulsive catching of breath
Pant *(verb)*
Puff *(noun)*
Wheeze *(verb)*
Heave *(verb)*

Gazebo *(noun)*–A small building, especially one in the garden of a house, that gives a wide view of the surrounding area
Summer house *(noun)*
Pavilion *(noun)*
Belvedere *(noun)*
Arbour *(noun)*

Generous *(adjective)*–Giving, big-hearted
Benevolent *(adjective)*
Charitable *(adjective)*
fair *(adjective)*
Thoughtful *(adjective)*

Gentle *(adjective)*–Having a mild or kind nature

Affable *(adjective)*
Amiable *(adjective)*
benign *(adjective)*
genial *(adjective)*

Giant *(adjective)*–Very large
Big *(adjective)*
Colossal *(adjective)*
Enormous *(adjective)*
Gigantic *(adjective)*

Glad *(adjective)*–Happy, delightful
Cheerful *(adjective)*
Contented *(adjective)*
Joyful *(adjective)*
Pleased *(adjective)*

Gloomy *(adjective)*–Dark, black
Bleak *(adjective)*
Dim *(adjective)*
dark *(adjective)*
Dismal *(adjective)*

Grant *(noun)*–Allowance, gift
Allocation *(noun)*
assistance *(noun)*
Award *(noun)*
Charity *(noun)*

Guilty *(adjective)*–Blameworthy, found at fault
Convicted *(adjective)*
Culpable *(adjective)*
Liable *(adjective)*
Responsible *(adjective)*

Good *(adjective)*–Pleasant, fine
    Excellent *(adjective)*
    Exceptional *(adjective)*
    Positive *(adjective)*
    Ace *(adjective)*

Give *(verb)* –Contribute, supply, transfer
    Allow *(verb)*
    Award *(verb)*
    Donate *(verb)*
    Permit *(verb)*

Glint *(noun)*–A small flash of light, especially a reflected one
    Glitter *(noun)*
    Gleam *(noun)*
    Sparkle *(noun)*
    Twinkle *(noun)*

Gobsmacked *(adjective)*–Utterly astounded
    Surprised *(adjective)*
    Startled *(adjective)*
    Amazed *(adjective)*
    Taken aback *(adjective)*

Gore *(noun)*–Blood that has been shed, especially as a result of violence
    Bloodshed *(noun)*
    Slaughter *(noun)*
    Carnage *(noun)*
    Butchery *(noun)*

Grime *(noun)*–Dirt engrained on the surface of something
    Smut *(noun)*
    Soot *(noun)*

H

Dust *(noun)*
Filth *(noun)*

Happy *(adjective)*–In high spirits
Cheerful *(adjective)*
Delighted *(adjective)*
Elated *(adjective)*
Joyous *(adjective)*

Hard *(adjective)*–Rocklike
Solid *(adjective)*
Strong *(adjective)*
Tough *(adjective)*
Compact *(adjective)*

Harmful *(adjective)*–Injurious, hurtful
Adverse *(adjective)*
bad *(adjective)*
damaging *(adjective)*
Destructive *(adjective)*

Harsh *(adjective)*–Rough, crude to the senses
Bitter *(adjective)*
Grim *(adjective)*
Rigid *(adjective)*
Severe *(adjective)*

Hate *(noun)*–Extreme dislike
Animosity *(noun)*
Antagonism *(noun)*
Enmity *(noun)*
Hatred *(noun)*

Healthy *(adjective)*–In good condition
Active *(adjective)*
Athletic *(adjective)*
Hearty *(adjective)*
Robust *(adjective)*

Hinder *(verb)* –Prevent, slow down
Block *(verb)*
Curb *(verb)*
Deter *(verb)*
Hamper *(verb)*

Humble *(adjective)*–Meek, unassuming
Courteous *(adjective)*
Modest *(adjective)*
Ordinary *(adjective)*
Shy *(adjective)*

Harangue *(noun)*–A lengthy and aggressive speech
Lecture *(noun)*
Tirade *(noun)*
Rant *(noun)*
Diatribe *(noun)*

Harbinger *(noun)*–A person or thing that announces or signals the approach of another
Herald *(noun)*
Signal *(noun)*
Indicator *(noun)*
Announcer *(noun)*

Haughtiness *(noun)*–The appearance or quality of being arrogantly

superior and disdainful
  Arrogance *(noun)*
  Pride *(noun)*
  Conceit *(noun)*
  Egotism *(noun)*

Hebetude *(noun)*–The state of being dull or lethargic
  Apathy *(noun)*
  Dullness *(noun)*
  Drowsiness *(noun)*
  Indolence *(noun)*

Hector *(verb)* –Talk to someone in a bullying way
  Intimidate *(verb)*
  Browbeat *(verb)*
  Badger *(verb)*
  Harass *(verb)*

Hedonism *(noun)*–The pursuit of pleasure
  Self-indulgence *(noun)*
  Epicureanism *(noun)*
  Self-gratification *(noun)*
  Overindulgence *(noun)*

Heretical *(adjective)*–Believing in or practicing religious heresy
  Dissident *(adjective)*
  Non-conformist *(adjective)*

Unorthodox *(adjective)*
Renegade *(adjective)*

Hitch *(noun)*–A temporary difficulty or problem
  Issue *(noun)*
  Snag *(noun)*
  Setback *(noun)*
  Hindrance *(noun)*

Hoary *(adjective)*–Overused and unoriginal
  Trite *(adjective)*
  Clichéd *(adjective)*
  Banal *(adjective)*
  Ordinary *(adjective)*

Hoi polloi *(noun)*–The common people
  The masses *(noun)*
  The crowd *(noun)*
  The populace *(noun)*
  The public *(noun)*

Hortative *(adjective)*–Giving strong encouragement
  Academic *(adjective)*
  Enlightening *(adjective)*
  Preachy *(adjective)*
  Sermonic *(adjective)*

Horde *(noun)*–A large group of people
  Crowd *(noun)*
  Mob *(noun)*

I

Swarm *(noun)*
Gathering *(noun)*

Illusory *(adjective)*–Based on illusion; not real
Whimsical *(adjective)*
Delusive *(adjective)*
Fallacious *(adjective)*
Fictitious *(adjective)*

Imbue *(verb)* –Inspire or permeate with a feeling or quality
Saturate *(verb)*
Diffuse *(verb)*
Suffuse *(verb)*
Pervade *(verb)*

Imbecility *(noun)*–Retardation more severe than a moron but not as severe as an idiot
Absurdity *(noun)*
Craziness *(noun)*
Stupidity *(noun)*
Imprudence *(noun)*

Impel *(verb)* –Drive, force or urge someone to do something
Exhort *(verb)*
Press *(verb)*
Incite *(verb)*
Persuade *(verb)*

Impetuosity *(noun)*–Rash impulsiveness
Brashness *(noun)*

Carelessness *(noun)*
Rashness *(noun)*
Temerity *(noun)*

Impiety *(noun)*–Lack of piety or reverance
Immorality *(noun)*
sacrilege *(noun)*
Disrespect *(noun)*
Vice *(noun)*

Important *(adjective)*–Valuable, substantial
Critical *(adjective)*
crucial *(adjective)*
Imperative *(adjective)*
Paramount *(adjective)*

Immense *(adjective)*–Extremely large
Boundless *(adjective)*
Endless *(adjective)*
Enormous *(adjective)*
Extensive *(adjective)*

Increase *(noun)*–Addition, growth
Boost *(noun)*
Escalation *(noun)*
Expansion *(noun)*
Increment *(noun)*

Inferior *(adjective)*–Less in rank, importance
Lesser *(adjective)*

Secondary *(adjective)*
Subordinate *(adjective)*
Menial *(adjective)*

Intelligent *(adjective)*–Very smart
Astute *(adjective)*
brilliant *(adjective)*
Wise *(adjective)*
Knowledgeable *(adjective)*

Interesting *(adjective)*–Appealing, entertaining
Attractive *(adjective)*
Intriguing *(adjective)*
Fascinating *(adjective)*
Engaging *(adjective)*

Internal *(adjective)*–Within
Domestic *(adjective)*
Private *(adjective)*
Inherent *(adjective)*
Innate *(adjective)*

Intentional *(adjective)*–Deliberate
Premeditated *(adjective)*
Willful *(adjective)*
calculated *(adjective)*
Considered *(adjective)*

Impugn *(verb)* –Dispute the truth or honesty of a statement or motive; call into question
Challenge *(verb)*
Query *(verb)*
Impeach *(verb)*
Take issue with *(verb)*

Impish *(adjective)*–Inclined to do slightly naughty things for fun
Mischievous *(adjective)*
Wicked *(adjective)*
Devilish *(adjective)*
Roguish *(adjective)*

Improvident *(adjective)*–Not having or showing foresight
Spendthrift *(adjective)*
Wasteful *(adjective)*
Extravagant *(adjective)*
Immoderate *(adjective)*

Implication *(noun)*–The conclusion that can be drawn from something although it is not explicitly stated
Inference *(noun)*
Insinuation *(noun)*
Intimation *(noun)*
Innuendo *(noun)*

Inadvertently *(adverb)* –Without intention
Accidentally *(adverb)*
Unintentionally *(adverb)*
Unwittingly *(adverb)*
Mistakenly *(adverb)*

Incunabulum *(noun)*–An early printed book, especially one printed before 1501
Inception *(noun)*
Beginning *(noun)*
Start *(noun)*
Outset *(noun)*

Inchoate *(adjective)*–Just begun and so not fully formed or developed
Rudimentary *(adjective)*
Amorphous *(adjective)*
Elementary *(adjective)*
Immature *(adjective)*

Incompliant *(adjective)*–Failing to act in accordance with a wish or command

Intransigent *(adjective)*
Mulish *(adjective)*
Headstrong *(adjective)*
Intractable *(adjective)*

Incriminate *(verb)* –Make someone appear guilty of a crime or wrongdoing
Implicate *(verb)*
Involve *(adjective)*
Allege *(adjective)*
Frame *(adjective)*

Inculpate *(verb)* –Accuse or blame
Incriminate *(adjective)*
Involve *(adjective)*
Implicate *(adjective)*
Accuse *(adjective)*

Indecorous *(adjective)*–Not in keeping with good taste and propriety
Improper *(adjective)*
Unseemly *(adjective)*
Indiscreet *(adjective)*
Immoral *(adjective)*

Infirmary *(noun)*–A hospital
Dispensary
Sickroom
Sick bay

Ingenerate *(adjective)*–To generate or produce within
Beget *(verb)*
Engender *(verb)*
Innate *(adjective)*
Inborn *(adjective)*

Ingress *(noun)*–The action or fact of going in or entering
Entry *(noun)*
Access *(noun)*
Admission *(noun)*

Approach *(noun)*

Ingratiating *(adjective)*–Intended to gain approval or favour
Sycophantic *(adjective)*
Fawning *(adjective)*
Servile *(adjective)*
Submissive *(adjective)*

Inhesion *(noun)*–The action or state of inhering in something
Adhesion *(noun)*
Incision *(noun)*
Invasion *(noun)*
Incursion *(noun)*

Inscrutable *(adjective)*–Impossible to understand or interpret
Enigmatic *(adjective)*
Unreadable *(adjective)*
Impenetrable *(adjective)*
Mysterious *(adjective)*

Insouciant *(adjective)*–Showing a casual lack of concern
Nonchalant *(adjective)*
Unruffled *(adjective)*
Frivolous *(adjective)*
Carefree *(adjective)*

Insolvency *(noun)*–The state of being insolvent
Bankruptcy *(noun)*
Liquidation *(noun)*
Ruination *(noun)*
Collapse *(noun)*

Instructive *(adjective)*–Useful and informative
Revealing *(verb)*
Explanatory *(adjective)*
Telling *(adjective)*
Instructional *(adjective)*

Insurgent *(noun)*–A person fighting against a government or invading force

Rebel *(noun)*
Revolutionary *(noun)*
Anarchist *(noun)*
Terrorist *(noun)*

Interplait *(verb)* –To plait together

Intertwine *(verb)*
Weave *(verb)*
Braid *(verb)*
Enmesh *(verb*

Interpolate *(verb)* –To insert into a conversation

Inject *(verb)*
Insert *(verb)*
Append *(verb)*
Interpose *(verb)*

Intransigent *(adjective)*–Unwilling or refusing to change one's views or to agree about something

Inflexible *(adjective)*
Unbending *(adjective)*
Stubborn *(adjective)*
Obstinate *(adjective)*

Intrigue *(verb)* –Arouse the curiosity or interest of

Fascinate *(verb)*
Draw *(verb)*
Tempt *(verb)*
Tantalize *(verb)*

Indictment *(noun)*–A formal charge or accusation of a serious crime

Citation *(noun)*
Allegation *(noun)*
Charge *(noun)*
Impeachment *(noun)*

Indomitable *(adjective)*–Impossible to subdue or defeat

Invincible *(adjective)*
Unconquerable *(adjective)*
Unbeatable *(adjective)*
Invulnerable *(adjective)*

Inoculable *(adjective)*– Susceptible to a disease transmitted by inoculation

Spreading *(adjective)*
Catching *(adjective)*
Infectious *(adjective)*
Transmissible *(adjective)*

Insolence *(noun)*–Rude and disrespectful behaviour

Impertinence *(noun)*
Impudence *(noun)*
Incivility *(noun)*
Discourtesy *(noun)*

Inwrought *(adjective)*–Intricately embroidered with a pattern or decoration

Intrinsic *(adjective)*
innate *(adjective)*
Inherent *(adjective)*
Ingrained *(adjective)*

Iota *(noun)*–An extremely small amount

Mite *(noun)*
Speck *(noun)*
Fraction *(noun)*
Morsel *(noun)*

Irascible *(adjective)*–Having or showing a tendency to be easily angered

Irritable *(adjective)*
Snappy *(adjective)*
Tetchy *(adjective)*
Waspish *(adjective)*

Irate *(adjective)*–Feeling or characterized by great anger

Furious *(adjective)*
Incensed *(adjective)*
Enraged *(adjective)*
Incandescent *(adjective)*

Iridescent *(adjective)*–Showing luminous colours that seem to change when seen from different angles

Glittering *(adjective)*
Sparkling *(adjective)*
Dazzling *(adjective)*
Lustrous *(adjective)*

Irrefutable *(adjective)*–Impossible to deny or disprove
Indisputable *(adjective)*

J

Unassailable *(adjective)*
Impregnable *(adjective)*
Indubitable *(adjective)*

Jaded *(adjective)*–Lacking enthusiasm, typically after having had too much of something
  Satiated *(verb)*
  Sated *(verb)*
  Bored *(adjective)*
  Gorged *(verb)*

Jamboree –A large celebration, typically a lavish and boisterous one
  Party *(noun)*
  Fiesta *(noun)*
  Gala *(noun)*
  Carnival *(noun)*

Jangle *(noun)*–A ringing metallic sound
  Clank *(noun)*
  Clash *(noun)*
  Rattle *(verb)*
  Clangour *(noun)*

Jaunt *(noun)*–A short journey made for pleasure
  Excursion *(noun)*
  Trip *(noun)*
  Expedition *(noun)*
  Holiday *(noun)*

Jiggle *(verb)* –Move about quickly from side to side or up and down
  Fidget *(verb)*
  Wriggle *(verb)*
  Squirm *(verb)*
  Shimmy *(verb)*

Jilt *(verb)* –Ssuddenly reject or abandon someone, especially a lover
  Dump *(verb)*
  Discard *(verb)*
  Desert *(verb)*
  Ditch *(verb)*

Jocular *(adjective)*–Said or done as a joke
  Jovial *(adjective)*
  Playful *(adjective)*
  Comical *(adjective)*
  Mischievous *(adjective)*

Join *(verb)* –Unite
  Add *(verb)*
  Adhere *(verb)*
  Affix *(verb)*
  Append *(verb)*

Just *(adjective)*–Fair, impartial
  Equitable *(adjective)*
  Decent *(adjective)*
  Ethical *(adjective)*
  Honest *(adjective)*

Justice *(noun)*–Lawfulness, fairness

Honesty *(noun)*

Integrity *(noun)*

Amends *(noun)*

Compensation *(noun)*

Josh *(verb)* –Tease someone in a playful way

Razz *(verb)*

Banter *(verb)*

Rib *(verb)*

Kid *(verb)*

K

Juggernaut *(noun)*–A large, heavy vehicle, especially an articulated lorry
Steamroller *(noun)*
Blitz *(noun)*
Barrage *(noun)*
Junket *(noun)*

Ken *(noun)*–One's range of knowledge or understanding
Awareness *(noun)*
Perception *(noun)*
Comprehension *(noun)*
Recognition *(noun)*

Keepsake *(noun)*–A small item kept in memory of the person who gave it or originally owned it
Memento *(noun)*
Souvenir *(noun)*
Memorial *(noun)*

Token *(noun)*

Keg *(noun)*–A small barrel, especially one of less than 10 gallons or *(in the US)* 30 gallons
Cask *(noun)*
Vat *(noun)*
Container *(noun)*
Vessel *(noun)*

Knead *(verb)* –Work into dough or paste with the hands
Form *(verb)*
Mold *(verb)*
Ply *(verb)*
Shape *(verb)*

Knotty *(adjective)*–Full of knots
Gnarled *(adjective)*
Complicated *(adjective)*
Convulated *(adjective)*
Tortuous *(adjective)*

L

Knowledge *(noun)*–Person's understanding; information
  Education *(noun)*
  Insight *(noun)*
  Learning *(noun)*
  Observation *(noun)*

Labile *(adjective)*–Liable to change
  Altered *(adjective)*

Labyrinth *(noun)*–A complicated irregular network of passages or paths in which it is difficult to find one's way
  Maze *(noun)*
  Web *(noun)*
  Coil *(noun)*
  Warren *(noun)*

Lace *(noun)*–A fine open fabric of cotton or silk, used especially for trimming garments
  Netting *(noun)*
  Tulle *(noun)*
  Mesh *(noun)*
  Webbing *(noun)*

Lacerate *(verb)* –Tear or deeply cut
  Gash *(verb)*
  Slash *(verb)*
  Rend *(verb)*
  Maul *(verb)*

Lackey *(noun)*–A servant, especially a manservant
  Flunkey *(noun)*
  Footman *(noun)*
  Steward *(noun)*
  Retainer *(noun)*

Laconic *(adjective)*–Using very few words
  Brief *(adjective)*
  Concise *(adjective)*
  Terse *(adjective)*
  Succinct *(adjective)*

Lackadaisical *(adjective)*–Lacking enthusiasm and determination
  Careless *(adjective)*
  Lax *(adjective)*
  Indifferent *(adjective)*
  Casual *(adjective)*

Lagger *(noun)*–Someone who lags behind
  Dawdler *(noun)*
  Idler *(noun)*
  Loafer *(noun)*
  Procrastinator *(noun)*

Laissez faire *(noun)*–The policy of leaving things to take their own course
  Indifference *(noun)*
  Free enterprise *(noun)*
  Neutrality *(noun)*
  Non-intervention *(noun)*

Laird *(noun)*–A person who owns a large estate in Scotland
  Landlord *(noun)*

Landowner *(noun)*
Proprietor *(noun)*
Retainer *(noun)*

Lama *(noun)*– A Tibetan or Mongolian Buddhist monk
Friar *(noun)*
Preacher *(noun)*
Holy man *(noun)*
Man of God *(noun)*

Lambent *(adjective)*– Glowing or flickering with a soft radiance
Bright *(adjective)*
Brilliant *(adjective)*
Lustrous *(adjective)*
Radiant *(adjective)*

Lament *(verb)* –A passionate expression of grief or sorrow
Howl *(verb)*
Wail *(verb)*
Moan *(verb)*
Sob *(verb)*

Lamina *(noun)*–A thin layer of sedimentary rock, organic tissue or other material
Coating *(noun)*
Film *(noun)*
Membrane *(noun)*
Parchment *(noun)*

Lampoon *(verb)* –Publicly criticise something or someone using sarcasm
Mock *(verb)*
Ridicule *(verb)*
Rag *(verb)*
Tease *(verb)*

Lamster *(adjective)*–A fugitive, especially from the law
Wanted *(adjective)*

Criminal *(adjective)*
Fleeting *(adjective)*
Elusive *(adjective)*

Landlubber *(noun)*–A person unfamiliar with the sea or sailing
Initiate *(noun)*
Tiro *(noun)*
Landsman *(noun)*
Novice *(noun)*

Lapidate *(verb)* –Kill by throwing stones at
Bombard *(verb)*
Hurl *(verb)*
Cast *(verb)*
Stone *(verb)*

Larceny *(noun)*–Theft of personal property
Robbery *(noun)*
Burglary *(noun)*
Purloining *(noun)*
Pilfering *(noun)*

Largesse *(noun)*–Generosity in bestowing gifts or money upon others
Munifience *(noun)*
Magnaminity *(noun)*
Lavishness *(noun)*
Benevolence *(noun)*

Lascivious *(adjective)*–Feeling or revealing an overt, sexual interest or desire
Lecherous *(adjective)*
Lewd *(adjective)*
Salacious *(adjective)*
Licentious *(adjective)*

Lass *(noun)*–a girl or young woman
Maid *(noun)*
Maiden *(noun)*
Damsel *(noun)*

Miss *(noun)*

Lave *(verb)* –Wash
Bathe *(verb)*
Rinse *(verb)*
Scour *(verb)*
Sponge *(verb)*

Latent *(adjective)*–A quality or state which is existing but not yet developed or manifest
Hidden *(adjective)*
Concealed *(adjective)*
Dormant *(adjective)*
Untapped *(adjective)*

Lattice *(noun)*–A structure made of wood or metal, used as a screen or fence or as a support for climbing plants
Grate *(noun)*
Grille *(noun)*
Trellis *(noun)*
Latticework *(noun)*

Launder *(verb)* –Wash and iron clothes
Cleanse *(verb)*
Clean *(verb)*
Do the laundry *(verb)*
Do the washing *(verb)*

Laud *(verb)* –Praise a person or their achievements highly
Extol *(verb)*
Applaud *(verb)*
Acclaim *(verb)*
Eulogise *(verb)*

Lagoon *(noun)*–A stretch of saltwater separated from the sea by a low sandbank or coral reef
Pond *(noun)*
Pool *(noun)*

Marsh *(noun)*
Shallows *(noun)*

Lacuna *(noun)*–An unfilled space
Gap *(noun)*
Cavity *(noun)*
Depression *(noun)*
Opening *(noun)*

Laxative *(noun)*–A medicine which facilitates evacuation of the bowels
Emetic *(noun)*
Aperitive *(noun)*
Cathartic *(noun)*
Purgative *(noun)*

Lazy *(adjective)*–Inactive, sluggish
Indifferent *(adjective)*
lethargic *(adjective)*
Idle *(adjective)*
Lagging *(adjective)*

Lend *(verb)* –Loan, accommodate
Contribute *(verb)*
Extend *(verb)*
Give *(verb)*
Advance *(verb)*

Lenient *(adjective)*–Permissive
Benign *(adjective)*
Forgiving *(adjective)*
Indulgent *(adjective)*
Tolerant *(adjective)*

Limited *(adjective)*–Restricted, definite
Defined *(adjective)*
Finite *(adjective)*
Narrow *(adjective)*
Bounded *(adjective)*

Loud *(adjective)*–Blaring, noisy
Boisterous *(adjective)*
Deafening *(adjective)*
Raucous *(adjective)*

Strident *(adjective)*

Loyal *(adjective)*–Faithful, dependable
Devoted *(adjective)*
Steadfast *(adjective)*
Trustworthy *(adjective)*
Dutiful *(adjective)*

Lea *(noun)*–An open area of grassy or arable land
Meadow *(noun)*
Acreage *(noun)*
Patch *(noun)*
Plot *(noun)*

Leaden *(adjective)*–Of the colour of lead; dull grey
Murky *(adjective)*
Gloomy *(adjective)*
Ashen *(adjective)*
Dark *(adjective)*

League *(noun)*–A collection of people or groups that combine for mutual protection or cooperation
Alliance *(noun)*
Confederation *(noun)*
Union *(noun)*
Coalition *(noun)*

Leafage *(noun)*–Leaf: the main organ of photosynthesis and transpiration in higher plants
Vegetation *(noun)*
Herbage *(noun)*
Verdure *(noun)*
Frondescence *(noun)*

Lectern *(noun)*–A tall stand with a sloping top to hold a book or notes, from which someone can read while standing up
Pulpit *(noun)*

Platform *(noun)*
Ambo *(noun)*
Rostrum *(noun)*

Levee *(noun)*–An embankment built to prevent the overflow of a river
Dam *(noun)*
Breakwater *(noun)*
Mound *(noun)*
Bank *(noun)*

Levity *(noun)*–The treatment of a serious matter with humour or lack of due respect
Gaiety *(noun)*
Fun *(noun)*
Hilarity *(noun)*
Glee *(noun)*

Lepidote *(adjective)*–Rough to the touch
Blotchy *(adjective)*
Scaly *(adjective)*
Scabby *(adjective)*
Encrusted *(adjective)*

Libertine *(noun)*–A person, especially a man, who freely indulges in sensual pleasures without regard to moral principles
Philanderer *(noun)*
Playboy *(noun)*
Rake *(noun)*
Lothario *(noun)*

Licentious *(adjective)*–Unprincipled in sexual matters
Promiscuous *(adjective)*
Debauched *(adjective)*
Degenerate *(adjective)*
Immoral *(adjective)*

Liege *(noun)*–A feudal superior or sovereign

Lord *(noun)*
Chieftain *(noun)*
Baron *(noun)*
Monarch *(noun)*

Librate *(verb)* –To oscillate or move from side to side or between two points
Lurch *(verb)*
Vacillate *(verb)*
Sway *(verb)*
Undulate *(verb)*

Lifer *(noun)*–A person sentenced to or serving a term of life imprisonment
Convict *(noun)*
Offender *(noun)*
Felon *(noun)*
Prisoner *(noun)*

Limpid *(adjective)*–Completely clear and transparent
Glassy *(adjective)*
Crystalline *(adjective)*
Translucent *(adjective)*
Unclouded *(adjective)*

Liturgy *(noun)*–A form or formulary according to which public religious worship, especially

Christian worship, is conducted
Rite *(noun)*
Ritual *(noun)*
Service *(noun)*
Sacrament *(noun)*

Locution *(noun)*–A word or phrase, especially with regard to style or idiom
Inflection *(noun)*
Dialect *(noun)*
Expression *(noun)*
Diction *(noun)*

Logomania *(noun)*–Pathologically excessive talking
Blarney *(noun)*
Talkative *(adjective)*
Flowing tongue *(noun)*
Gift of the gab *(noun)*

Lofty *(adjective)*–Of imposing height
Tall *(adjective)*
High *(adjective)*
Giant *(adjective)*
Towering *(adjective)*

Lord *(noun)*–A man of noble rank or high office
Peer *(noun)*

M

Aristocrat *(noun)*
Patrician *(noun)*
Grandee *(noun)*

Lorgnons *(noun)*–An eyeglass or a pair of eyeglasses
Monocle *(noun)*
Pince-nez *(noun)*

Maceration *(verb)* –Softening due to soaking
Steeping *(verb)*
Susurration *(verb)*
Undertone *(noun)*
Mollescence *(noun)*

Machismo *(noun)*–Strong or aggressive masculine pride
Macho *(adjective)*
Chauvinism *(noun)*
Sexism *(noun)*
Manliness *(noun)*

Mad *(adjective)*–Crazy, insane
Delirious *(adjective)*
Demented *(adjective)*
Nutty *(adjective)*
Psychotic *(adjective)*

Malicious *(adjective)*–Hateful
Malevolent *(adjective)*
Malignant *(adjective)*
Nasty *(adjective)*
Vicious *(adjective)*

Mature *(adjective)*–Adult, grown-up

Cultivated *(adjective)*
Cultured *(adjective)*
Grown *(adjective)*
Ready *(adjective)*

Maximum *(adjective)*–Highest, utmost
Best *(adjective)*
Superlative *(adjective)*
Ultimate *(adjective)*
Paramount *(adjective)*

Messy *(adjective)*–Cluttered, dirty
Chaotic *(adjective)*
Confused *(adjective)*
Sloppy *(adjective)*
careless *(adjective)*

Minority *(noun)*–An outnumbered group
Less than half *(noun)*
Splinter group *(noun)*
The outvoted *(noun)*
Opposition *(noun)*

Miser *(noun)*–Person who hoards money, possessions
Cheapskate *(noun)*
Hoarder *(noun)*
Tightwad *(noun)*
Pinchpenny *(noun)*

Misunderstand *(verb)* –Get the wrong idea
Misconstrue *(verb)*

Misinterpret *(verb)*
Misjudge *(verb)*
Misread *(verb)*

Maelstrom *(noun)*–A powerful whirlpool in the sea or river
Turbulence *(noun)*
Vortex *(noun)*
Eddy *(noun)*
Swirl *(noun)*

Magnum *(noun)*–Holder for physical object
Box *(noun)*
Carton *(noun)*
Crate *(noun)*
Vessel *(noun)*

Manoeuvre *(verb)* –A movement or series of moves requiring skill and care
Operation *(verb)*
Exercise *(verb)*
Activity *(verb)*
Action *(verb)*

Maven *(noun)*–Someone who is at the top of his/her respective field expert *(noun)*
Connoisseur *(noun)*
Judge *(noun)*
Arbitrator *(noun)*

Minutiae *(noun)*–The small precise or trivial details of something
Niceties *(noun)*
Subtleties *(noun)*
Particulars *(noun)*
Specifics *(noun)*

Missive *(noun)*–A letter, especially a long or official one
Memorandum *(noun)*
Report *(noun)*
Notification *(noun)*

Dispatch *(noun)*

Melee *(noun)*–A confused fight or scuffle
Rumpus *(noun)*
Commotion *(noun)*
Disorder *(noun)*
Disturbance *(noun)*

Meridian *(noun)*–A point or period of highest development, prosperity, etc
Acme *(noun)*
Apex *(noun)*
Crest *(noun)*
Peak *(noun)*

Milieu *(noun)*–A person's social environment
Background *(noun)*
Setting *(noun)*
Habitat *(noun)*
Domain *(noun)*

Moccasin *(noun)*–A soft leather slipper or shoe
Slipper *(noun)*
Sandal *(noun)*
Shoe *(noun)*

Moil *(verb)* –Hard work
Drudge *(verb)*
Grind *(verb)*
Toil *(verb)*
Struggle *(verb)*

Moniker *(noun)*–A name
Tag *(noun)*
Handle *(noun)*
Label *(noun)*
Denominatio *(noun)*

Moppet *(noun)*–A small endearingly sweet child
Child *(noun)*
Toddler *(noun)*
Kid *(noun)*

Tyke *(noun)*

Mordant *(adjective)*–Having a sharp or critical sense of humour

  Caustic *(adjective)*

  Trenchant *(adjective)*

  Acerbic *(adjective)*

Scathing *(adjective)*

Multitude *(noun)*–A large number of people or things

  Horde *(noun)*

  Mass *(noun)*

  Abundance *(noun)*

N

Profusion *(noun)*

Muffle *(verb)* –Cover or wrap up a source of sound to reduce its loudness
  Hush *(verb)*
  Mute *(verb)*
  Muzzle *(verb)*
  Stifle *(verb)*

Narrow *(adjective)*–Confined, restricted
  Cramped *(adjective)*
  Limited *(adjective)*
  Compressed *(adjective)*
  Confining *(adjective)*

Neat *(adjective)*–Arranged well, uncluttered
  Immaculate *(adjective)*
  Orderly *(adjective)*
  Precise *(adjective)*
  Tidy *(adjective)*

Noisy *(adjective)*–Very loud and unharmonious in sound

Boisterous *(adjective)*
Cacophonous *(adjective)*
Rowdy *(adjective)*
Vociferous *(adjective)*

Naught *(noun)*–Nothing
  Nought *(noun)*
  Nil *(noun)*
  Zero *(noun)*
  Zilch *(noun)*

Neoteric *(adjective)*–Belonging to recent times
  Modern *(adjective)*
  Newborn *(adjective)*
  Current *(adjective)*
  Contemporary *(adjective)*

Nostrum *(noun)*–A medicine prepared by an unqualified person, especially one that is not considered effective
  Potion *(noun)*
  Elixir *(noun)*

O

Panacea *(noun)*
Cure-all *(noun)*

Noxious *(adjective)*–Very unpleasant
Poisonous *(adjective)*
Toxic *(adjective)*
Deadly *(adjective)*
Virulent *(adjective)*

Oaf *(noun)*–A man who is rough or clumsy and unintelligent
Lout *(noun)*
Boor *(noun)*
Clown *(noun)*
Bumpkin *(noun)*

Oasis *(noun)*–A fertile spot in a desert, where water is found
Watering hole *(noun)*
Watering place *(noun)*
Spring *(noun)*
Claypan *(noun)*

Obdurate *(adjective)*–Stubbornly refusing to change one's opinion or course of action
Adamant *(adjective)*
Dogged *(adjective)*
Implacable *(adjective)*
Obstinate *(adjective)*

Obedient *(adjective)*–Well-behaved, submissive
Compliant *(adjective)*
Deferential *(adjective)*

Devoted *(adjective)*
Faithful *(adjective)*

Optimist *(noun)*–Positive thinker
Dreamer *(noun)*
Idealist *(noun)*
Hoper *(noun)*
Pollyanna *(noun)*

Obeisance *(noun)*–Deferential respect
Homage *(noun)*
Reverance *(noun)*
Submission *(noun)*
Deferance *(noun)*

Obelisk *(noun)*–A tapering stone pillar, typically having a square or rectangular cross section, set up as a monument or landmark
Column *(noun)*
Monolith *(noun)*
Memorial *(noun)*
Shaft *(noun)*

Obfuscate *(verb)* –Make obscure, unclear or unintelligible
Confuse *(verb)*
Muddle *(verb)*
Garble *(verb)*
Cloud *(verb)*

Objurgate *(verb)* –Rebuke severely
Scold *(verb)*

Chide *(verb)*
Reprimand *(verb)*
Reproach *(verb)*

Obituary *(noun)*–A notice of a death, especially in a newspaper, typically including a brief biography of the deceased person
Eulogy *(noun)*
Death notice *(noun)*
Obit *(noun)*
Announcement *(noun)*

Oblation *(noun)*–A thing presented or offered to a God
Sacrifice *(noun)*
Presentation *(noun)*
Gift *(noun)*
Offering *(noun)*

Oblivious *(adjective)*–Not aware of or concerned about what is happening around one
Heedless *(adjective)*
Ignorant *(adjective)*
Unsuspecting *(adjective)*
Impervious *(adjective)*

Obliteration *(noun)*–The action or fact of total destruction
Removal *(noun)*
Eradication *(noun)*
Extermination *(noun)*
Demolition *(noun)*

Obloquy *(noun)*–Strong public condemnation
Vilification *(noun)*
Defamation *(noun)*
Invective *(noun)*
Libel *(noun)*

Oblong *(adjective)*–A rectangular object or flat figure with unequal adjacent sides
Oval *(adjective)*
Elliptical *(adjective)*
Egg-shaped *(adjective)*
Ovate *(adjective)*

Oboe *(noun)*–A woodwind instrument with a double-reed mouthpiece, a slender tubular body, and holes stopped by keys
Horn *(noun)*
Pipe *(noun)*
Clarinet *(noun)*
Flute *(noun)*

Obsequious *(adjective)* –Obedient or attentive to an excessive degree
Servile *(adjective)*
Ingratiating *(adjective)*
Sycophantic *(adjective)*
Fawning *(adjective)*
Subservient *(adjective)*

Observant *(adjective)*–Quick to notice things
Alert *(adjective)*
Attentive *(adjective)*
Watchful *(adjective)*
Vigilant *(adjective)*

Obsolete *(adjective)*–Out of date; no longer used
Outdated *(adjective)*
Outmoded *(adjective)*
Antiquated *(adjective)*
Discontinued *(adjective)*

Obstreperous *(adjective)*–Noisy and difficult to control
Boisterous *(adjective)*
Loud *(adjective)*
Rambunctious *(adjective)*
Rowdy *(adjective)*

Obvallate *(verb)*–To surround with, or as with, a wall
  Walled-up *(adjective)*
  Walled-in *(noun)*
  Sealed-up *(adjective)*

Obverse *(noun)*–The opposite of a fact or truth
  Counterpart *(noun)*
  Complement *(noun)*
  Face *(noun)*
  Front *(noun)*

Obviate *(verb)* –Remove a need or difficulty
  Preclude *(verb)*
  Prevent *(verb)*
  Remove *(verb)*
  Avert *(verb)*

Ochre *(adjective)*–An earthy pigment containing ferric oxide, typically with clay, varying from light yellow to brown or red
  Fawn *(adjective)*
  Mahogony *(adjective)*
  Tan *(adjective)*
  Tawny *(adjective)*

Octave *(noun)*–A series of eight notes occupying the interval between two notes
  Note *(noun)*
  Scale *(noun)*
  Tone *(noun)*
  Interval *(noun)*

Occult *(noun)*–Magical powers, practices or phenomena
  Witchcraft *(noun)*
  Sorcery *(noun)*
  Necromancy *(noun)*

Mysticism *(noun)*

Ode *(noun)*–A lyric poem, typically one in the form of an address to a particular subject
  Sonnet *(noun)*
  Ballad *(noun)*
  Poesy *(noun)*
  Rhyme *(noun)*

Odious *(adjective)*–Extremely unpleasant
  Repulsive *(adjective)*
  Revolting *(adjective)*
  Disgusting *(adjective)*
  Deplorable *(adjective)*

Odium *(noun)*–General or widespread hatred or disgust incurred by someone as a result of their actions
  Abhorrence *(noun)*
  Loathing *(noun)*
  Aversion *(noun)*
  Contempt *(noun)*

Odoriferous *(adjective)* Having or giving off a distinctive smell
  Pungent *(adjective)*
  Savoury *(adjective)*
  Balmy *(adjective)*
  Redolent *(adjective)*

Odyssey *(noun)*–A long, wandering and eventful journey
  Trek *(noun)*
  Expedition *(noun)*
  Quest *(noun)*
  Sojourn *(noun)*

Offbeat *(adjective)*–Unusual or unconventional
  Unorthodox *(adjective)*
  Strange *(adjective)*

Idiosyncratic *(adjective)*
Quirky *(adjective)*

Off-colour *(adjective)*–Slightly in-decent
Obscene *(adjective)*
Smutty *(adjective)*
Crude *(adjective)*
Filthy *(adjective)*

Offender *(noun)*–A person who commits an illegal act
Criminal *(noun)*
Felon *(noun)*
Delinquent *(noun)*
Culprit *(noun)*

Offhand *(adjective)*–Ungraciously or offensively non-chalant or cool in manner
Indifferent *(adjective)*
casual *(adjective)*
Aloof *(adjective)*
Cavalier *(adjective)*

Offal *(noun)*–The entrails and in-ternal organs of an animal used as food
Carrion *(noun)*
Remains *(noun)*
Fragments *(noun)*
Dregs *(noun)*

Officious *(adjective)*–Assertive of authority in a domineering way, es-pecially with regard to trivial mat-ters
Self-important *(adjective)*
Dictatorial *(adjective)*
Interfering *(adjective)*
Opinionated *(adjective)*

Officiate *(verb)*–Act as an official in charge of something
Manage *(verb)*
Oversee *(verb)*
Supervise *(verb)*
Conduct *(verb)*

Offset *(verb)*–Counteract some-thing by having an equal and op-posite force or effect
Counterbalance *(verb)*
Neutralise *(verb)*
Nullify *(verb)*
Counterpoise *(verb)*

Offspring *(noun)*–A person's child or children
Progeny *(noun)*
Youngsters *(noun)*
Brood *(noun)*
Infants *(noun)*

Ogre *(noun)*–A man-eating giant in folklore
Monster *(noun)*
Giant *(noun)*
Troll *(noun)*
Bogeyman *(noun)*

Oligarchy *(noun)*–A small group of people having control of a coun-try or organisation
Autocracy *(noun)*
Domination *(noun)*
Despotism *(noun)*
Totalitarianism *(noun)*

Omnibus *(noun)*–A volume con-taining several books previously published separately
Compilation *(noun)*
Anthology *(noun)*
Vehicle *(noun)*
Whole *(noun)*

Omniscient *(adjective)*–Knowing everything
    Wise *(adjective)*
    Knowledgeable *(adjective)*
    Pre-eminent *(adjective)*
    All-seeing *(adjective)*

Omneity *(noun)*–That which is all-pervading or all-comprehensive
    Absoluteness *(noun)*
    Completeness *(noun)*
    Aggregate *(noun)*
    Ensemble *(noun)*

Onerous *(adjective)*–Involving a great deal of effort
    Troublesome *(adjective)*
    Difficult *(adjective)*
    Burdensome *(adjective)*
    Inconvenient *(adjective)*

Oncoming *(adjective)*–Approaching from the front
    Advancing *(adjective)*
    Coming *(adjective)*
    Arriving *(adjective)*
    Onrushing *(adjective)*

Onslaught *(noun)*–A fierce or destructive attack
    Assault *(noun)*
    Offensive *(noun)*
    Charge *(noun)*
    Storming *(noun)*

Onus *(noun)*–Something that is one's duty or responsibility
    Burden *(noun)*
    Liability *(noun)*
    Obligation *(noun)*
    Encumbrance *(noun)*

Opera *(noun)*–A dramatic work in one or more acts, set to music for singers and instrumentalists
    Opus *(noun)*
    Production *(noun)*
    Composition *(noun)*
    Oeuvre *(noun)*

Opportune *(adjective)*–Convenient or appropriate time for a particular action or event
    Auspicious *(adjective)*
    Favourable *(adjective)*
    Advantageous *(adjective)*
    Providential *(adjective)*

Opulent *(adjective)*–Ostentatiously costly and luxurious
    Sumptuous *(adjective)*
    Lavish *(adjective)*
    Magnificent *(adjective)*
    Grand *(adjective)*

Opiate *(noun)*–A drug derived from or related to opium
    Narcotic *(noun)*
    Sedative *(noun)*
    Tranquiliser *(noun)*
    Depressant *(noun)*

Oppressive *(adjective)*–Inflicting harsh treatment
    Brutal *(adjective)*
    Repressive *(adjective)*
    Tyrannical *(adjective)*
    Despotic *(adjective)*

Opprobrious *(adjective)*–Expressing scorn or criticism
    Abusive *(adjective)*
    Derogatory *(adjective)*
    Disparaging *(adjective)*
    Offensive *(adjective)*

Oracle *(noun)*–A priest or priest-

ess acting as a medium through whom advice or prophecy was sought from the Gods in classical antiquity
  Edict *(noun)*
  Vision *(noun)*
  Revelation *(noun)*
  Divination *(noun)*

Oration *(noun)*–A formal speech, especially one given on a ceremonial occasion
  Address *(noun)*
  Lecture *(noun)*
  Sermon *(noun)*
  Discourse *(noun)*

Ordain *(verb)* –Make someone a priest or minister
  Appoint *(verb)*
  Induct *(verb)*
  Anoint *(verb)*
  Consecrate *(verb)*

Ordeal *(noun)*–A very unpleasant and prolonged experience
  Trial *(noun)*
  Tribulation *(noun)*
  Trauma *(noun)*
  Torment *(noun)*

Ordination *(noun)*–The action of ordaining someone in holy orders
  Appointment *(noun)*
  Consecration *(noun)*
  Installation *(noun)*
  Investiture *(noun)*

Organic *(adjective)*–Relating to or derived from living matter
  Animate *(adjective)*
  Biological *(adjective)*
  Natural *(adjective)*
  Biotic *(adjective)*

Orient *(verb)* –Align or position something relative to the points of a compass or other specified positions
  Place *(verb)*
  Dispose *(verb)*
  Situate *(verb)*
  Set *(verb)*

Orb *(noun)*–A spherical object or shape
  Sphere *(noun)*
  Globe *(noun)*
  Ball *(noun)*
  Circle *(noun)*

Ordinance *(noun)*–An authoritative order
  Edict *(noun)*
  Decree *(noun)*
  Law *(noun)*
  Injunction *(noun)*

Ordnance *(noun)*–Mounted guns; artillery
  Cannon *(noun)*
  Arms *(noun)*
  Weapons *(noun)*
  Munitions *(noun)*

Orison *(noun)*–A prayer
  Appeal *(noun)*
  Benediction *(noun)*
  Petition *(noun)*
  Plea *(noun)*

Orts *(noun)*–Scraps; remains
  Fraction *(noun)*
  Fragment *(noun)*
  Mite *(noun)*
  Particle *(noun)*

Ossify *(verb)* –Turn into bone or bony tissue
   Harden *(verb)*
   Solidify *(verb)*
   Stiffen *(verb)*
   Petrify *(verb)*

Ossuary *(noun)*–A container or room in which the bones of dead people are placed
   Urn *(noun)*
   Receptacle *(noun)*
   Vault *(noun)*
   Vessel *(noun)*

Ostensibly *(adverb)* –As appears or is stated to be true
   Apparently *(adverb)*
   Seemingly *(adverb)*
   Outwardly *(adverb)*
   Superficially *(adverb)*

Ounce *(noun)*–A very small amount of something
   Scrap *(noun)*
   Speck *(noun)*
   Whit *(noun)*
   Fragment *(noun)*

Oust *(verb)* –Drive out or expel someone from a position or place
   Remove *(verb)*
   Eject *(verb)*
   Depose *(verb)*
   Unseat *(verb)*

Outbreak *(noun)*–A sudden occurrence of something unwelcome, such as war or disease
   Eruption *(noun)*
   Upsurge *(noun)*
   Outburst *(noun)*
   Epidemic *(noun)*

Outclass *(verb)* –Be far superior to
   Surpass *(verb)*
   Outshine *(verb)*
   Overshadow *(verb)*
   Eclipse *(verb)*

Outlast *(verb)* –Live or last longer than
   Outlive *(verb)*
   Survive *(verb)*
   Weather *(verb)*
   Outwear *(verb)*

Outlying *(adjective)*–Situated far from a centre
   Remote *(adjective)*
   Distant *(adjective)*
   Faraway *(adjective)*
   Peripheral *(adjective)*

Outpost *(noun)*–A remote station
   Frontier *(noun)*
   Settlement *(noun)*
   Boundary *(noun)*

Outrageous *(adjective)*–Shockingly bad or excessive
   Disgraceful *(adjective)*
   Scandalous *(adjective)*
   Appalling *(adjective)*
   Abhorrent *(adjective)*

Outrun *(verb)* –Run or travel faster or further than
   Outstrip *(verb)*
   Outdistance *(verb)*
   Outpace *(verb)*
   Overtake *(verb)*

Outré *(adjective)*–Unusual and typically rather shocking
   Weird *(adjective)*
   Queer *(adjective)*
   Grotesque *(adjective)*
   Eccentric *(adjective)*

Outmoded *(adjective)*–Old-fashioned
  Outdated *(adjective)*
  Archaic *(adjective)*
  Antiquated *(adjective)*
  Obsolete *(adjective)*

Outrage *(noun)*–An extremely strong reaction of anger, shock or indignation
  Rage *(noun)*
  Wrath *(noun)*
  Horror *(noun)*
  Disgust *(noun)*

Outrageous *(adjective)*–Shockingly bad or excessive
  Disgraceful *(adjective)*
  Scandalous *(adjective)*
  Atrocious *(adjective)*
  Heinous *(adjective)*

Outright *(adjective)*–Open and direct
  Absolute *(adjective)*
  Thorough *(adjective)*
  Categorical *(adjective)*
  Consummate *(adjective)*

Outspoken *(adjective)*–Frank in stating one's opinions
  Forthright *(adjective)*
  Direct *(adjective)*
  Candid *(adjective)*
  Honest *(adjective)*

Outwardly *(adverb)* –On the surface
  Apparently *(adverb)*
  Superficially *(adverb)*
  Ostensibly *(adverb)*
  Evidently *(adverb)*

Outwit *(verb)* –Deceive by greater ingenuity
  Outsmart *(verb)*
  Outmanoeuvre *(verb)*
  Outplay *(verb)*
  Trick *(verb)*

Overall *(adjective)*–Taking everything into account
  General *(adjective)*
  Comprehensive *(adjective)*
  Universal *(adjective)*
  Gross *(adjective)*

Overawe *(verb)* –Impress someone so much that they are silent or inhibited
  Intimidate *(verb)*
  Daunt *(verb)*
  Awe *(verb)*
  Disconcert *(verb)*

Overcast *(adjective)*–Marked by a covering of grey cloud; dull
  Cloudy *(adjective)*
  Leaden *(adjective)*
  Murky *(adjective)*
  Foggy *(adjective)*

Overcharge *(verb)* –Charge someone to high a price for goods or a service
  Swindle *(verb)*
  Cheat *(verb)*
  Defraud *(verb)*
  Fleece *(verb)*

Overpass *(noun)*–A bridge by which a road or railway line passes over another
  Footbridge *(noun)*
  Walkway *(noun)*
  Skyway *(noun)*
  Span *(noun)*

Overrule *(verb)* –Reject or disallow by exercising one's superior authority

Countermand *(verb)*
Rescind *(verb)*
Override *(verb)*
Veto *(verb)*

Overhaul *(verb)* –Take apart a piece of machinery in order to examine and repair it

Service *(verb)*
Repair *(verb)*
Mend *(verb)*
Maintain *(verb)*

Overlord *(noun)*–A ruler, especially a feudal lord

Chief *(noun)*
Emperor *(noun)*
Ruler *(noun)*
Suzerain *(noun)*

Overshot *(verb)* –To omit or avoid

Skip *(verb)*
Evade *(verb)*
Leave *(verb)*
Miss *(verb)*

Oversight *(noun)*–An unintentional failure to notice or do something

Omission *(noun)*
Lapse *(noun)*
Slip *(noun)*
Miscalculation *(noun)*

Overwrought *(adjective)*–In a state of nervous excitement or anxiety

Tense *(adjective)*
Agitated *(adjective)*
Edgy *(adjective)*
Jittery *(adjective)*

Overture *(noun)*–An introduction to something more substantial

Prelude *(noun)*
Precursor *(noun)*
Forerunner *(noun)*
Harbinger *(noun)*

Overt *(adjective)*–Done or shown openly

Plain *(adjective)*
Clear *(adjective)*
Apparent *(adjective)*
Obvious *(adjective)*

Overtone *(noun)*–A subtle or subsidiary quality

Connotation *(noun)*
Implication *(noun)*
Hint *(noun)*
Suggestion *(noun)*

Overweening *(adjective)*–Showing excessive confidence or pride

Conceited *(adjective)*
Smug *(adjective)*
Arrogant *(adjective)*

P

Proud *(adjective)*

Oxymoron *(noun)*–A figure of speech in which apparently contradictory terms appear in conjunction
    Antithesis *(noun)*
    Parable *(noun)*
    Device *(noun)*
    Conceit *(noun)*

Paean *(noun)*–A song of praise or triumph
    Hymn *(noun)*
    Ode *(noun)*
    Psalm *(noun)*
    Anthem *(noun)*

Palliation *(verb)* –Easing the severity of a pain or a disease without removing the cause
    Alleviation *(verb)*
    Assuagement *(verb)*
    Ease *(verb)*
    Reprieve *(verb)*

Pall *(noun)*–A dark cloud of smoke, dust, etc
    Cloak *(noun)*
    mantle *(noun)*
    Veil *(noun)*
    Shroud *(noun)*

Panegyric *(noun)*–A public speech or published text in praise of someone or something

Eulogy *(noun)*
Accolade *(noun)*

Parlay *(verb)* –Turn an initial stake or winnings from a previous bet into a greater amount
    Gamble *(verb)*
    Speculate *(verb)*
    Venture *(verb)*
    Wager *(verb)*

Pariah *(noun)*–An outcast
    Reject *(noun)*
    Untouchable *(noun)*
    Undesirable *(noun)*
    Unwanted *(noun)*

Parlance *(noun)*–A particular way of speaking or using words
    Jargon *(noun)*
    Lingo *(noun)*
    Vernacular *(noun)*
    Expression *(noun)*

Patient *(adjective)*–Willing to endure
    Calm *(adjective)*
    Tolerant *(adjective)*
    Forgiving *(adjective)*
    Understanding *(adjective)*

Peace *(noun)*–Harmony, agreement
    Accord *(noun)*
    Truce *(noun)*
    Amity *(noun)*
    Concord *(noun)*

Permanent *(adjective)*–Constant, lasting
>Durable *(adjective)*
>Enduring *(adjective)*
>Perpetual *(adjective)*
>Stable *(adjective)*

Plentiful *(adjective)*–Abundant
>Ample *(adjective)*
>Bountiful *(adjective)*
>Generous *(adjective)*
>Prolific *(adjective)*

Polite *(adjective)*–Mannerly, civilised
>Affable *(adjective)*
>Civil *(adjective)*
>Cordial *(adjective)*
>Courteous *(adjective)*

Poverty *(noun)*–Want; extreme need, often financial
>Hardship *(noun)*
>Lack *(noun)*
>Scarcity *(noun)*
>Dearth *(noun)*

Powerful *(adjective)*–Strong, effective
>Dominant *(adjective)*
>Forceful *(adjective)*
>Mighty *(adjective)*
>Potent *(adjective)*

Pretty *(adjective)*–Attractive
>Beautiful *(adjective)*
>Charming *(adjective)*
>Lovely *(adjective)*
>Appealing *(adjective)*

Private *(adjective)*–Personal, intimate
>Confidential *(adjective)*
>Secret *(adjective)*
>Exclusive *(adjective)*
>Privy *(adjective)*

Prudent *(adjective)*–Wise, sensible in action and thought
>Careful *(adjective)*
>cautious *(adjective)*
>Discreet *(adjective)*
>Shrewd *(adjective)*

Pure *(adjective)*–Unmixed, genuine
>Authentic *(adjective)*
>Natural *(adjective)*
>Real *(adjective)*
>True *(adjective)*

Patrimony *(noun)*–Property inherited from one's father or male ancestor
>Endowment *(noun)*
>Estate *(noun)*
>Heritage *(noun)*
>Legacy *(noun)*

Pedantry *(noun)*–Excessive concern with minor details and rules
>Dogmatism *(noun)*
>Purism *(noun)*
>Literalism *(noun)*
>Formalism *(noun)*

Perfidious *(adjective)*–Deceitful and untrustworthy
>Treacherous *(adjective)*
>Duplicitous *(adjective)*
>Traitorous *(adjective)*
>False *(adjective)*

Perchance *(adverb)*–By some chance; perhaps
>Mayhap *(adverb)*
>Feasible *(adjective)*

Could be *(adverb)*
Might be *(adverb)*

Perfidy *(noun)*–The state of being deceitful and untrustworthy
Treachery *(noun)*
Duplicity *(noun)*
Betrayal *(noun)*
Treason *(noun)*

Perpetuity *(noun)*–The state or quality of lasting forever
Continuity *(noun)*
Constancy *(noun)*
Continuance *(noun)*
Endurance *(noun)*

Pejorative *(adjective)*–Expressing contempt or disapproval
Disparaging *(adjective)*
Insulting *(adjective)*
Slanderous *(adjective)*
Derogatory *(adjective)*

Perfunctory *(adjective)*–An action which is carried out without any real interest
Cursory *(adjective)*
Desultory *(adjective)*
Token *(adjective)*
Casual *(adjective)*

Phantasmagoria *(noun)*–A sequence of real or imaginary images like that seen in a dream
Phantom *(noun)*
Apparition *(noun)*
Wraith *(noun)*
Illusion *(noun)*

Phizog *(noun)*–A person's face or expression
Demeanor *(noun)*

Visage *(noun)*
Aspect *(noun)*
Mien *(noun)*

Phlegmatic *(adjective)*–Having an unemotional and calm disposition
Apathetic *(adjective)*
Dispassionate *(adjective)*
Frigid *(adjective)*
Indifferent *(adjective)*

Piquant *(adjective)*–Having a pleasantly sharp taste or appetizing flavour
Spicy *(adjective)*
Tangy *(adjective)*
Savoury *(adjective)*
Tart *(adjective)*

Polyglot *(noun)*–Knowing or using several languages
Linguist *(noun)*
Glossator *(noun)*
Cryptographer *(noun)*
Dragoman *(noun)*

Polemics *(noun)*–A strong verbal or written attack on someone or something
Diatribe *(noun)*
Invective *(noun)*
Harangue *(noun)*
Denunciation *(noun)*

Portent *(noun)*–A sign or warning that a momentous or calamitous is likely to happen
Omen *(noun)*
Sign *(noun)*
Indication *(noun)*
Signal *(noun)*

Posit *(verb)* –Put forward as fact or as a basis for argument
Postulate *(verb)*

Propound *(verb)*
Hypothesize *(verb)*
Predicate *(verb)*

Platitudes *(noun)*–A remark or statement, especially one with a moral content, that has been used too often to be interesting or thoughtful
Cliché *(noun)*
Truism *(noun)*
Commonplace *(noun)*
Banality *(noun)*

Pliable *(adjective)*–Easily bent; flexible
Elastic *(adjective)*
Supple *(adjective)*
Pliant *(adjective)*
Malleable *(adjective)*

Plutocrat *(noun)*–A person whose power derives from their wealth
capitalist *(noun)*
Tycoon *(noun)*
Magnate *(noun)*
Nouveau riche *(noun)*

Pragmatism *(noun)*–A pragmatic attitude or policy
Appropriateness *(noun)*
Aptness *(noun)*
Effectiveness *(noun)*
Suitability *(noun)*

Precedent *(noun)*–An earlier event or action that is regarded as an example to be considered in subsequent similar circumstances
Model *(noun)*
Pattern *(noun)*
Standard *(noun)*
Yardstick *(noun)*

Priggish *(adjective)*–Self-righteous-ly moralistic and superior
Sanctimonious *(adjective)*
Prudish *(adjective)*
Prim *(adjective)*
Prissy *(adjective)*

Prior *(adjective)*–Existing or coming before in time, or importance
Previous *(adjective)*
Foregoing *(adjective)*
Antecedent *(adjective)*
Preliminary *(adjective)*

Proclivity *(noun)*–A tendency to choose or do something regularly
Propensity *(noun)*
Penchant *(noun)*
Leaning *(noun)*
Preference *(noun)*

Progenitor *(noun)*–A person or thing from which a person, animal or plant is descended
Ancestor *(noun)*
Forefather *(noun)*
Forebear *(noun)*
Parent *(noun)*

Profligate *(adjective)*–Recklessly extravagant or wasteful in the use of resources
Improvident *(adjective)*
Immoderate *(adjective)*
Excessive *(adjective)*
Reckless *(adjective)*

Pronouncement *(noun)*–A formal or authoritative announcement or declaration
Proclamation *(noun)*
Judgement *(noun)*
Ruling *(noun)*

Decree *(noun)*

Propound *(verb)* –Put forward an idea or theory for consideration by others

    Advance *(verb)*

    Offer *(verb)*

    Present *(verb)*

    Submit *(verb)*

Prance *(verb)* –Move with high springy steps

    Gambol *(verb)*

    Bound *(verb)*

    Jump *(verb)*

Leap *(verb)*

Puritanical *(adjective)*–Having or displaying a very strict moral attitude towards self-indulgence or sex

    Moralistic *(adjective)*

    Stuffy *(adjective)*

    Starchy *(adjective)*

    Prudish *(adjective)*

Purvey *(verb)* –Provide or supply food, drink or other goods as one's business

    Furnish *(verb)*

    Cater *(verb)*

Q

Retail *(verb)*
Trade *(verb)*

Pusillanimous *(adjective)*–Showing a lack of courage or determination
Timid *(adjective)*
Afraid *(adjective)*
Cowardly *(adjective)*
Tame *(adjective)*

Qualified *(adjective)*–Able, skillful
Accomplished *(adjective)*
Capable *(adjective)*
Competent *(adjective)*
Experienced *(adjective)*

Quiet *(adjective)*–Without or with little sound
Soft *(adjective)*
Silent *(adjective)*
Peaceful *(adjective)*
Hushed *(adjective)*

Qualmish *(verb)* –A sudden feeling of sickness, faintness or nausea
Sickly *(verb)*
Squeamish *(verb)*
Nauseated *(verb)*
Unwell *(verb)*

Quandary *(noun)*–A state of uncertainty over what to do in a difficult situation

Dilemma *(noun)*
Plight *(noun)*
Predicament *(noun)*
Perplexity *(noun)*

Quell *(verb)* –Put an end to something, typically by the use of force
Finish *(verb)*
Crush *(verb)*
Suppress *(verb)*
Thwart *(verb)*

Quill *(noun)*–Any of the main wing or tail feathers of a bird
Plumage *(noun)*
Plume *(noun)*
Down *(noun)*
Pinion *(noun)*

Quisling *(noun)*–A traitor who collaborates with an enemy force occupying their country
Collaborator *(noun)*
Sympathiser *(noun)*
Fraterniser *(noun)*
Colluder *(noun)*

Quixotic *(adjective)*–Extremely idealistic; unrealistic and impractical
Romantic *(adjective)*
Utopian *(adjective)*

R

Perfectionist *(adjective)*
Unworldly *(adjective)*

Quotidian *(adjective)*–Of or occurring everyday
Daily *(adjective)*
Usual *(adjective)*
Trivial *(adjective)*
Commonplace *(adjective)*

Raise *(noun)*–Increase in salary or position
Boost *(noun)*
Hike *(noun)*
Increment *(noun)*
Bump *(noun)*

Rapid *(adjective)*–Very quick
Accelerated *(adjective)*
Fast *(adjective)*
Hasty *(adjective)*
Speedy *(adjective)*

Rare *(adjective)*–Exceptional
Extraordinary *(adjective)*
Scarce *(adjective)*
Uncommon *(adjective)*
Unique *(adjective)*

Regular *(adjective)*–Normal, common
Daily *(adjective)*
Ordinary *(adjective)*
Typical *(adjective)*

Usual *(adjective)*

Real *(adjective)*–Genuine in existence
Actual *(adjective)*
Authentic *(adjective)*
Original *(adjective)*
True *(adjective)*

Rich *(adjective)*–Having a lot of money
Affluent *(adjective)*
prosperous *(adjective)*
Wealthy *(adjective)*
Flush *(adjective)*

Rough *(adjective)*–Uneven, irregular
Choppy *(adjective)*
Coarse *(adjective)*
Harsh *(adjective)*
Rugged *(adjective)*

Rude *(adjective)*–Disrespectful, rough
Boorish *(adjective)*
Crude *(adjective)*
Impolite *(adjective)*
Surly *(adjective)*

Rancorous *(adjective)*–Characterized by bitterness or resentment
Spiteful *(adjective)*
Hateful *(adjective)*

Rampart → Repose

Malicious *(adjective)*
Malevolent *(adjective)*

Rambunctious *(adjective)*–Uncontrollably exuberant
Boisterous *(adjective)*
Noisy *(adjective)*
Unruly *(adjective)*
Rowdy *(adjective)*

Rampart *(noun)*–A defensive wall of a castle or walled city
Battlement *(noun)*
Embankment *(noun)*
Fortification *(noun)*
Bastion *(noun)*

Rebuke *(verb)* –Express sharp disapproval of someone because of their behaviour or actions
Reprimand *(verb)*
Admonish *(verb)*
Castigate *(verb)*
Berate *(verb)*

Rebuff *(verb)* –Reject someone or something in an abrupt or ungracious manner *(verb)*
Spurn *(verb)*
Refuse *(verb)*
Decline *(verb)*
Repudiate *(verb)*

Recompense *(verb)* –Make amends to someone for loss or harm suffered
Compensate *(verb)*
Repay *(verb)*
Reimburse *(verb)*
Indemnify *(verb)*

Recondite *(adjective)*–A little known subject or knowledge
Abstruse *(adjective)*
Obscure *(adjective)*

Abstract *(adjective)*
Arcane *(adjective)*

Reconnaissance *(noun)*–Military observation of a region to locate an enemy or ascertain strategic features
Survey *(verb)*
Exploration *(verb)*
Inspection *(verb)*
Probe *(verb)*

Recuperate *(verb)* –Having the effect of restoring health or strength
Recover *(verb)*
Restore *(verb)*

Recusant *(noun)*–A person who refuses to submit to an authority or to comply with a regulation
Hostile *(noun)*
Opposed *(noun)*
Dissident *(noun)*
Nonconformist *(noun)*

Redolent *(adjective)*–Strongly reminiscent of
Evocative
Suggestive
Reminiscent
Remindful

Remonstrate *(verb)* –Make a forcefully reproachful protest
Complain *(verb)*
Expostulate *(verb)*
Reprimand *(verb)*
Reprehend *(verb)*

Relegate *(verb)* –Assign an inferior rank or position to
Downgrade *(verb)*
Lower *(verb)*
Demote *(verb)*
Degrade *(verb)*

Repast *(noun)*–A meal

Feast *(noun)*
banquet *(noun)*
Snack *(noun)*
Spread *(noun)*

Repose *(noun)*–A state of rest, sleep or tranquility
Relaxation *(noun)*
Inactivity *(noun)*
Idleness *(noun)*
Slumber *(noun)*

Repository *(noun)*–A place where things may be stored
Archive *(noun)*
Safe *(noun)*
Stockroom *(noun)*
Vault *(noun)*

Reprehensible *(adjective)*–Deserving censure or condemnation
Deplorable *(adjective)*
Disgraceful *(adjective)*
Wrong *(adjective)*
Despicable *(adjective)*

Reproach *(noun)*–The expression of disapproval or disappointment
Rebuke *(noun)*
Reproof *(noun)*
Admonition *(noun)*
Scolding *(noun)*

Repine *(verb)* –Feel or express discontent
Fret *(verb)*
Mope *(verb)*
Languish *(verb)*
Brood *(verb)*

Repugnance *(noun)*–Intense disgust
Revulsion *(noun)*
Abhorrence *(noun)*
Loathing *(noun)*
Hatred *(noun)*

Renegade *(adjective)*–Having treacherously changed alliance
Traitorous *(adjective)*
Disloyal *(adjective)*
Mutinous *(adjective)*
Perfidious *(adjective)*

Rescind *(verb)* –Revoke, cancel or repeal a law, order or agreement
Overturn *(verb)*
Overrule *(verb)*
Annul *(verb)*
Nullify *(verb)*

Resplendent *(adjective)*–Attractive and impressive through being richly colourful or sumptuous
Splendid *(adjective)*
Magnificent *(adjective)*
Brilliant *(adjective)*
Dazzling *(adjective)*

Roister *(verb)* –Enjoy oneself or celebrate in a noisy or boisterous way
Revel *(verb)*
carouse *(verb)*
Frolic *(verb)*
Romp *(verb)*

Romp *(verb)* –Play roughly and energetically
Frolic *(verb)*
frisk *(verb)*
Gambol *(verb)*
Prance *(verb)*

Roving *(verb)* –Travel constantly without a fixed destination
Wander *(verb)*
Roam *(verb)*
Ramble *(verb)*
Drift *(verb)*

Rumpus *(noun)*–A noisy disturbance; a row

S

Commotion *(noun)*
Uproar *(noun)*
Furore *(noun)*
Ruckus *(noun)*

Ruse *(noun)*–An action intended to deceive someone
Trick *(noun)*
Ploy *(noun)*
tactic *(noun)*
Scheme *(noun)*

Safe *(adjective)*–Free from harm
Intact *(adjective)*
protected *(adjective)*
Secure *(adjective)*
Okay *(adjective)*

Satisfactory *(adjective)*–Acceptable, sufficient
Adequate *(adjective)*
Gratifying *(adjective)*
Solid *(adjective)*
Appeasing *(adjective)*

Secure *(adjective)*–Safe
Protected *(adjective)*
Defended *(adjective)*
Guarded *(adjective)*
Sheltered *(adjective)*

Scatter *(verb)* –Strew, disperse
Spread *(verb)*
Sprinkle *(verb)*
Distribute *(verb)*

Fling *(verb)*

Serious *(adjective)*–Somber, humourless
Severe *(adjective)*
Sincere *(adjective)*
Sober *(adjective)*
Austere *(adjective)*

Shallow *(adjective)*–Not deep
Empty *(adjective)*
Hollow *(adjective)*
Trifling *(adjective)*
Depthless *(adjective)*

Shrink *(verb)* –Become smaller
Decrease *(verb)*
Diminish *(verb)*
Dwindle *(verb)*
Reduce *(verb)*

Sick *(adjective)*–Not healthy, not feeling well
Ailing *(adjective)*
Ill *(adjective)*
Indisposed *(adjective)*
Invalid *(adjective)*

Simple *(adjective)*–Clear, understandable; easy
Elementary *(adjective)*
Plain *(adjective)*
Uncomplicated *(adjective)*
Incomplex *(adjective)*

Sink *(verb)* –Fall in, go under
  Capsize *(verb)*
  Descend *(verb)*
  Drown *(verb)*
  Plummet *(verb)*

Sorrow *(noun)*–Extreme upset, grief
  Agony *(noun)*
  Anguish *(noun)*
  Misery *(noun)*
  sadness *(noun)*

Strict *(adjective)*–Authoritarian
  Draconian *(adjective)*
  Harsh *(adjective)*
  Severe *(adjective)*
  Stern *(adjective)*

Success *(noun)*–Favourable outcome
  Accomplishment *(noun)*
  Achievement *(noun)*
  Triumph *(noun)*
  Victory *(noun)*

Sweltering *(adjective)*–Very hot
  Baking *(adjective)*
  Oppressive *(adjective)*
  Scorching *(adjective)*
  Sultry *(adjective)*

Sashay *(verb)* –Walk in an ostentatious yet casual manner
  Flounce *(verb)*
  Glide *(verb)*
  Strut *(verb)*
  Swagger *(verb)*

Sartorial *(adjective)*–Relating to tailoring, clothes or style of dress
  Stylistic *(adjective)*
  Elegant *(adjective)*
  Impeccable *(adjective)*
  Trim *(adjective)*

Scion *(noun)*–A descendent of a notable family
  Offshoot *(noun)*
  Heir *(noun)*
  Issue *(noun)*
  Offspring *(noun)*

Scourge *(noun)*–A person or thing that causes great trouble or suffering
  Affliction *(noun)*
  Bane *(noun)*
  Curse *(noun)*
  Menace *(noun)*

Scorn *(noun)*–A feeling and expression of contempt or disdain for someone or something
  Derision *(noun)*
  Mockery *(noun)*
  Ridicule *(noun)*
  Disdain *(noun)*

Scoff *(verb)* –Speak to someone or about something in a scornfully derisive or mocking way
  Ridicule *(verb)*
  Dismiss *(verb)*
  Taunt *(verb)*
  Tease *(verb)*

Scree *(noun)*–A mass of small loose stones that form or cover a slope on a mountain
  Rubble *(noun)*
  Sediment *(noun)*
  Shavings *(noun)*
  Grains *(noun)*

Sedulous *(adjective)*–Showing dedi-cation and diligence
  Meticulous *(adjective)*
  Assiduous *(adjective)*
  Attentive *(adjective)*
  Industrious *(adjective)*

Sequacious *(adjective)*–Lacking in-

dependence or originality of thought
    Compliant *(adjective)*
    Obedient *(adjective)*
    Servile *(adjective)*
    Subservient *(adjective)*

Shackles *(noun)*–A metal link, used to secure a chain or rope to something
    Handcuff *(noun)*
    Fetter *(noun)*
    Manacle *(noun)*
    Irons *(noun)*

Shenanigan *(verb)* –Reckless or malicious behaviour that causes discomfort or annoyance in others
    Gag *(verb)*
    Antic *(verb)*
    Joke *(verb)*
    Lark *(verb)*

Siege *(noun)*–A military operation in which enemy forces surround a town or building
    Blockade *(noun)*
    Besiege *(noun)*
    Put upon *(verb)*
    Set upon *(verb)*

Skewer *(noun)*–A long piece of wood or metal used for holding pieces of food, typically meat, together during cooking
    Brochette *(noun)*
    Lance *(noun)*
    Pin *(noun)*
    Truss *(noun)*

Slush *(noun)*–Partially melted snow or ice
    Mire *(noun)*
    Sludge *(noun)*
    Slosh *(noun)*
    Slop *(noun)*

Sojourn *(noun)*–A temporary stay
    Stopover *(noun)*
    Layover *(noun)*
    Rest *(noun)*
    Vacation *(noun)*

Solicitude *(noun)*–Care or concern for someone or something
    Mindfulness *(noun)*
    Consideration *(noun)*
    Thoughtfulness *(noun)*
    Worry *(noun)*

Solecism *(noun)*–A grammatical mistake in speech or writing
    Error *(noun)*
    Blunder *(noun)*
    Cacology *(noun)*
    Misusage *(noun)*

Subterfuge *(noun)*–Deceit used in order to achieve one's goal
    Trickery *(noun)*
    Intrigue *(noun)*
    Evasion *(noun)*
    Duplicity *(noun)*

Subaltern *(noun)*–Of lower status
    Assistant *(noun)*
    Inferior *(noun)*
    Subordinate *(noun)*

Sublessee *(noun)* A person who holds a sublease
    Occupant *(noun)*
    Boarder *(noun)*
    leaseholder *(noun)*
    Rentee *(noun)*

Surfeit *(noun)*–An excessive amount of something
    Surplus *(noun)*
    Abundance *(noun)*
    Glut *(noun)*

Superfluity *(noun)*

Surly *(adjective)*–Bad-tempered and unfriendly
Grumpy *(adjective)*
Glum *(adjective)*
Irascible *(adjective)*
Ungracious *(adjective)*

Scabrous *(adjective)*–Rough and covered with, or as if with, scabs
Blotchy *(adjective)*
Encrusted *(adjective)*
Scabby *(adjective)*
Scaly *(adjective)*

Scamper *(verb)* –Run with quick, light steps, especially through fear and excitement
Scurry *(verb)*
Scuttle *(verb)*
Dash *(verb)*
Sprint *(verb)*

Scraggy *(adjective)*–A person or animal who is thin and bony
Scrawny *(adjective)*
Skinny *(adjective)*
Gaunt *(adjective)*
Angular *(adjective)*

Schism *(noun)*–A split or division between strongly opposed sections or parties, caused by differences in opinion or belief
Rift *(noun)*
Breach *(noun)*
Severance *(noun)*
Estrangement *(noun)*

Semaphore *(noun)*–A system of sending messages by holding the arms or two flags or two poles in certain positions according to an al-phabetic code
Communicate *(verb)*
Gesticulate *(verb)*
Sign *(verb)*
Gesture *(verb)*

Sine qua non *(noun)* An essential condition, a thing that is absolutely necessary
Must *(noun)*
Necessity *(noun)*
Need *(noun)*
Prerequisite *(noun)*

Squirt *(verb)* –Cause a liquid to be ejected from a small opening in a thin fast stream
Spurt *(verb)*
jet *(verb)*
Spray *(verb)*
Spritz *(verb)*

Squeal *(noun)*–A long, high-pitched cry or noise
Screech *(verb)*
Scream *(verb)*
Shriek *(verb)*
Howl *(verb)*

Spectre *(noun)*–A ghost
Phantom *(noun)*
Apparition *(noun)*
Spirit *(noun)*
Wraith *(noun)*

Snare *(noun)*–A trap for catching birds or mammals
Gin *(noun)*
Net *(noun)*
Noose *(noun)*
Springe *(noun)*

Snoop *(noun)*–A furtive investiga-tion
Search *(verb)*

Prowl *(verb)*
Ferret *(verb)*
Exploration *(verb)*

Strident *(adjective)*–Loud and harsh sound
Raucous *(adjective)*
Grating *(adjective)*
Jarring *(adjective)*
Shrill *(adjective)*

Stymie *(verb)* –Prevent or hinder the progress of
Impede *(verb)*
Hamper *(verb)*
Obstruct *(verb)*
Thwart *(verb)*

Suffragist *(noun)*–A person advocating the extension of suffrage, especially to women
Citizen *(noun)*
Resident *(noun)*
Taxpayer *(noun)*
Balloter *(noun)*

Sylvan *(adjective)*–Consisting of or associated with woods
Wooded *(adjective)*
Rustic *(adjective)*
Shady *(adjective)*
Forestlike *(adjective)*

Svelte *(adjective)*–A slender and elegant person
Graceful *(adjective)*
Lissom *(adjective)*
Willowy *(adjective)*
Lean *(adjective)*

Swaggering *(verb)* –Walk or behave in a very confident and arrogant way
Strut *(verb)*

parade *(verb)*
Stride *(verb)*
Prance *(verb)*

Sweepstakes *(noun)*–A form of gambling, especially on horse races, in which all the stakes are divided among the winners
Stake *(noun)*
Wager *(noun)*
Lottery *(noun)*
Pot *(noun)*

Swerve *(verb)* –Change or cause to change direction abruptly
Veer *(verb)*
deviate *(verb)*
Diverge *(verb)*
Weave *(verb)*

Swelter *(verb)* –Be uncomfortably hot
Humid *(verb)*
Steamy *(verb)*
Sultry *(verb)*
Muggy *(verb)*

Swig *(verb)* –Drink in large draughts
Gulp *(verb)*
Guzzle *(verb)*
Swallow *(verb)*
Glug *(verb)*

Stein *(noun)*–A large earthenware beer mug
Vessel *(noun)*
Dish *(noun)*
Bowl *(noun)*
Jar *(noun)*

Strewn *(verb)* –Scatter or spread things untidily over a surface or area

Disperse *(verb)*
Litter *(verb)*
Toss *(verb)*
Sprinkle *(verb)*

Steeplechase *(noun)*–A horse race run on a racecourse having ditches and hedges as jumps
Game *(noun)*
Sporting *(noun)*
Field sport *(noun)*

Pursuit *(noun)*

Stupefaction *(noun)*–The state of being stupefied
Oblivion *(noun)*
Numbness *(noun)*
Unconsciousness *(noun)*
Insensibility *(noun)*

Swill *(verb)* –Drink something greedily or in large quantities
Quaff *(verb)*

T

Swallow *(verb)*
Guzzle *(verb)*
Drain *(verb)*

Synod *(noun)*–A Presbyterian ecclesiastical court above the presbyteries and subject to the General Assembly
    Assembly *(noun)*
    Body *(noun)*
    Convocation *(noun)*
    Committee (*noun*)

Tabernacle *(noun)*–A fixed or movable place of worship, typically of light construction
    Sanctuary *(noun)*
    Shrine *(noun)*
    Temple *(noun)*
    Reliquary *(noun)*

Tableau *(noun)*–A group of models or motionless figres representing a scene from a story or from history
    Picture *(noun)*
    Painting *(noun)*
    Representation *(noun)*
    Illustration *(noun)*

Tankard *(noun)*–A tall beer mug, typically made of silver or pewter, with a handle and sometimes a hinged lid

Flask *(noun)*
Flagon *(noun)*
Stoup *(noun)*
Cup *(noun)*

Tantamount *(adjective)*–Equivalent in seriousness to; virtually the same as
    Amounting to *(adjective)*
    As good as *(adjective)*
    More or less *(adjective)*
    Synonymous with *(adjective)*

Trope *(noun)*–A figurative or metaphorical use of a word or expression
    Allegory *(noun)*
    Allusion *(noun)*
    Metaphor *(noun)*
    Analogy *(noun)*

Taciturn *(adjective)*–Person who is reserved or uncommunicative in speech
    Reticent *(adjective)*
    Unforthcoming *(adjective)*
    Inarticulate *(adjective)*
    Unresponsive *(adjective)*

Tall *(adjective)*–High in stature, length
    Soaring *(adjective)*
    Towering *(adjective)*
    Big *(adjective)*

Great *(adjective)*
Tame *(adjective)*–domesticated, compliant
    Docile *(adjective)*
    Gentle *(adjective)*
    Mild *(adjective)*
    Subdued *(adjective)*

Thick *(adjective)*–Deep, bulky
    Chunky *(adjective)*
    Massive *(adjective)*
    Solid *(adjective)*
    Broad *(adjective)*

Tight *(adjective)*–Close, snug
    Compact *(adjective)*
    Cramped *(adjective)*
    Rigid *(adjective)*
    Strained *(adjective)*

Tiny *(adjective)*–Very small
    Miniature *(adjective)*
    Minuscule *(adjective)*
    Microscopic *(adjective)*
    Slight *(adjective)*

Tough *(adjective)*–Sturdy, strong
    Hard *(adjective)*
    resilient *(adjective)*
    Hardy *(adjective)*
    Stout *(adjective)*

Transparent *(adjective)*–See-through
    Clear *(adjective)*
    Thin *(adjective)*
    Translucent *(adjective)*
    Filmy *(adjective)*

Truth *(noun)*–Reality, validity
    Accuracy *(noun)*
    certainty *(noun)*
    Fact *(noun)*
    Actuality *(noun)*

Tardy *(adjective)*–Delaying or delayed beyond the right or expected time
    Overdue *(adjective)*
    Behind *(adjective)*
    Dawdling *(adjective)*
    Procrastinating *(adjective)*

Tautology *(noun)*–The saying of the same thing twice over in different words
    Repetition *(noun)*
    Redundancy *(noun)*
    Iteration *(noun)*
    Duplication *(noun)*

Tapestry *(noun)*–A piece of thick textile fabric with pictures or designs formed by weaving coloured weft threads or by embroidering on canvas, used as a wall hanging or soft furnishing
    Drapery *(noun)*
    Arras *(noun)*
    Dosser *(noun)*
    Hanging *(noun)*

Tenebrous *(adjective)*–Shadowy or obscure
    Dark *(adjective)*
    Dingy *(adjective)*
    Dusky *(adjective)*
    Gloomy *(adjective)*

Tenor *(noun)*–A singing voice between a baritone and alto or countertenor, the highest of the ordinary adult male range
    Tone *(noun)*
    Scale *(noun)*
    Note *(noun)*
    Scope *(noun)*

Termagant *(noun)*–A harsh-tempered or overbearing woman
    Fractious *(adjective)*
    Intemperate *(adjective)*
    Stormy *(adjective)*
    Uncompliant *(adjective)*

Tome *(noun)*–A book, especially a large, heavy, scholarly one
    Volume *(noun)*
    Work *(noun)*
    Opus *(noun)*
    Title *(noun)*

Torrential *(adjective)*–Rain falling rapidly and in copious quantities
    Severe *(adjective)*
    Heavy *(adjective)*
    Relentless *(adjective)*
    Downpour *(adjective)*

Thrall *(noun)*–The state of being in someone's power
    Control *(noun)*
    Grip *(noun)*
    Clutches *(noun)*
    Grasp *(noun)*

Tomfoolery *(noun)*–Foolish or silly behaviour
    Antics *(noun)*
    Nonsense *(noun)*
    Mischief *(noun)*
    Stupidity *(noun)*

Traducement *(noun)*–A false accusation or a malicious misrepresentation of someone's words or actions
    Aspersion *(noun)*
    Defamation *(noun)*
    Smear *(noun)*
    Denigration *(noun)*

Trenchant *(adjective)*–Vigorous or incisive in expression or style
    Cutting *(adjective)*
    Pointed *(adjective)*
    Piercing *(adjective)*
    Acute *(adjective)*

Transcendent *(adjective)*–Beyond or above the range of normal or physical human experience
    Abstract *(adjective)*
    Fantastic *(adjective)*
    Supernatural *(adjective)*
    Hypothetical *(adjective)*

U

Transmogrify *(verb)* –Transform in a surprising or magical manner
  Alter *(verb)*
  Interchange *(verb)*
  Metamorphose *(verb)*
  Mutate *(verb)*

Triage *(noun)*–The assignment of degrees of urgency to wounds or illnesses to decide the order of treatment of a large number of patients or casualties
  Sort *(noun)*
  Prioritise *(noun)*
  Methosise *(noun)*
  Systemise *(noun)*

Uberty *(noun)*–Readiness to bear, produce
  Abundance *(noun)*
  Fertility *(noun)*
  Copiousness *(noun)*
  Fruitfulness *(noun)*

Ubiety *(noun)*–The condition of being in a definite place
  Existence *(noun)*
  Being *(noun)*
  Subsistence *(noun)*
  Inhabitance *(noun)*

Ubiquity *(noun)*–The state of being everywhere at once
  Pervasiveness *(noun)*
  Universality *(noun)*
  All-presence *(noun)*

  Omnipresence *(noun)*

Uberous *(adjective)*–Ready to bear, produce
  Abundant *(adjective)*
  Fruitful *(adjective)*
  Fecund *(adjective)*
  Bountiful *(adjective)*

Ulcer *(noun)*–An open sore on an external or internal surface of the body
  Abscess *(noun)*
  Carbuncle *(noun)*
  Cyst *(noun)*
  Blister *(noun)*

Ulterior *(adjective)*–Existing beyond what is obvious or admitted
  Secondary *(adjective)*
  Underlying *(adjective)*
  Unapparent *(adjective)*
  Undisclosed *(adjective)*

Ultimatum *(noun)*–A final demand or statement of terms, the rejection of which will result in a breakdown in relations
  Warning *(noun)*
  Conditions *(noun)*
  Final proposal *(noun)*
  Final terms *(noun)*

Ultramarine *(noun)*–A brilliant deep blue pigment originally obtained

from lapis lazuli
Turquoise *(adjective)*
Azure *(adjective)*
Cerulean *(adjective)*
Cobalt *(adjective)*

Umber *(noun)*–A natural pigment resembling but darker than ochre, normally dark yellowish-brown in colour
Brick *(noun)*
Copper *(adjective)*
Rust *(adjective)*
Tawny *(adjective)*

Umbra *(noun)*–The fully shaded inner region of a shadow cast by an opaque object, especially the area on the earth or moon experiencing the total phase of an eclipse
Cover *(noun)*
Screen *(noun)*
Shadow *(noun)*
Obscurity *(noun)*

Umbrageous *(adjective)*–Filled with shade
Cloudy *(adjective)*
Screened *(adjective)*
Indistinct *(adjective)*
Shadowy *(adjective)*

Unabashed *(adjective)*–Not embarrassed, disconcerted, or ashamed
Brazen *(adjective)*
Audacious *(adjective)*
Immodest *(adjective)*
Flagrant *(adjective)*

Unabated *(adjective)*–Without any reduction in intensity or strength
Incessant *(adjective)*

Persistent *(adjective)*
Sustained *(adjective)*
Unrelenting *(adjective)*

Unaccustomed *(adjective)*–Not familiar or usual; out of the ordinary
Unusual *(adjective)*
Unfamiliar *(adjective)*
New *(adjective)*
Atypical *(adjective)*

Unassuming *(adjective)*–Not pretentious or arrogant
Modest *(adjective)*
Reserved *(adjective)*
Humble *(adjective)*
Meek *(adjective)*

Unavailing *(adjective)*–Achieving little or nothing
Ineffective *(adjective)*
Ineffectual *(adjective)*
Futile *(adjective)*
Unproductive *(adjective)*

Unbeaten *(adjective)*–Not defeated or surpassed
Unconquered *(adjective)*
Unbowed *(adjective)*
Unrivalled *(adjective)*
Unbroken *(adjective)*

Unbecoming *(adjective)*–Not flattering especially clothing or a colour
Unattractive *(adjective)*
Unsightly *(adjective)*
Hideous *(adjective)*
Ugly *(adjective)*

Unbridled *(adjective)*–Uncontrolled
Unconstrained *(adjective)*

Unrestrained *(adjective)*
Uninhibited *(adjective)*
Rampant *(adjective)*

Uncanny *(adjective)*–Strange or mysterious, especially in an unsettling way
Eerie *(adjective)*
Preternatural *(adjective)*
Bizarre *(adjective)*
Supernatural *(adjective)*

Uncivil *(adjective)*–Discourteous
Impolite *(adjective)*
Rude *(adjective)*
Insulting *(adjective)*
Impertinent *(adjective)*

Unconformity *(noun)*–A surface of contact between two groups of unconformable strata
Aberration *(noun)*
Abnormality *(noun)*
Deviation *(noun)*
Oddity *(noun)*

Unconscionable *(adjective)*–Not right or reasonable
Unethical *(adjective)*
Amoral *(adjective)*
Unprincipled *(adjective)*
Wrong *(adjective)*

Unconventionality *(noun)*–Originality by virtue of being unconventional
Idiosyncracy *(noun)*
Quirk *(noun)*
Peculiarity *(noun)*
Foible *(noun)*

Uncompromising *(adjective)*–
Showing an unwillingness to make concessions to others
Inflexible *(adjective)*
Obstinate *(adjective)*
Rigid *(adjective)*
Unbending *(adjective)*

Undeceive *(verb)* –Tell someone that an idea or belief is mistaken
Disillusion *(verb)*
Disenthrall *(verb)*
Disentranced *(verb)*

Underhand *(adjective)*–Acting or done in a secret or dishonest way
Deceitful *(adjective)*
Dishonest *(adjective)*
Immoral *(adjective)*
Dubious *(adjective)*

Underling *(noun)*–A person lower in status or rank
Subordinate *(noun)*
Inferior *(noun)*
Lackey *(noun)*
menial *(noun)*

Underpass *(noun)*–A road or pedestrian tunnel passing under a road or railway
Passage *(noun)*
crossway *(noun)*
Crosswalk *(noun)*
Intersection *(noun)*

Underrate *(verb)* –Underestimate the extent, value or importance of someone or something
Undervalue *(verb)*
Downgrade *(verb)*
reduce *(verb)*
lessen *(verb)*

Underscore *(noun)*–A line drawn under a word or phrase for emphasis

Highlight
Stress
Accentuate
Indicate

Underside *(noun)*–The bottom or lower side or surface of something
Belly *(noun)*
Root *(noun)*
Sole *(noun)*
Underneath *(noun)*

Undersigned *(noun)*–Person who has signed a letter or document
Endorser *(noun)*
Petitioner *(noun)*
Signatory *(noun)*
Subscriber *(noun)*

Understate *(verb)* –Describe or represent somethingas being less good or important than it really is
Downplay *(verb)*
Underrate *(verb)*
Underplay *(verb)*
Trivialise *(verb)*

Understudy *(noun)*–A person who learns another's role in the theatre in order to be able to act at short notice in their absence
Substitute *(noun)*
Replacement *(noun)*
Proxy *(noun)*
Standby *(noun)*

Undertaker *(noun)*–A person whose business is preparing dead bodies for burial or cremation and making arrangements for funerals
Funeral director *(noun)*
Mortician *(noun)*
Embalmer *(noun)*

Grave digger *(noun)*

Undertow *(noun)*–Undercurrent
Eddy *(noun)*
Vortex *(noun)*
Whirlpool *(noun)*
Riptide *(noun)*

Univocal *(adjective)*–Having only one possible meaning
Unambiguous *(adjective)*
Absolute *(adjective)*
Categorical *(adjective)*
Obvious *(adjective)*

Unrestrained *(adjective)*–Not restrained or restricted
Uncontrolled *(adjective)*
Unchecked *(adjective)*
Unfettered *(adjective)*
Unshackled *(adjective)*

Unction *(noun)*–The action of anointing someone with oil or ointment as a religious rite or as a symbol of investiture as a monarch
Chrism *(noun)*
Lotion *(noun)*
Salve *(noun)*
Unguent *(noun)*

Uncurl *(verb)* –Straighten or cause to straighten from a curled position
Uncoil *(verb)*
Unravel *(verb)*
Align *(verb)*
Level *(verb)*

Unfettered *(adjective)*–Not confined or restricted
Unrestrained *(adjective)*
Unconstrained *(adjective)*
Unbound *(adjective)*
Unimpeded *(adjective)*

Ungula *(noun)*–Nail of an animal; tool shaped like the nail of an animal
    Paw *(noun)*
    Pincer *(noun)*
    Talon *(noun)*
    Grappler *(noun)*

Undulant *(adjective)*–Having a rising and falling motion or appearance like that of waves
    Lurching *(adjective)*
    Rolling *(adjective)*
    Waving *(adjective)*
    Rippling *(adjective)*

Undercroft *(noun)*–The crypt of a church
    Grotto *(noun)*
    Catacomb *(noun)*
    Vault *(noun)*
    Mausoleum *(noun)*

Unsafe *(adjective)*–Dangerous
    Hazardous *(adjective)*
    Perilous *(adjective)*
    Risky *(adjective)*
    Unreliable *(adjective)*

Useful *(adjective)*–Beneficial, valuable
    Advantageous *(adjective)*
    Effective *(adjective)*
    Convenient *(adjective)*
    Favourable *(adjective)*

Untenable *(adjective)*–A position or view which is not able to be maintained or defended against attack or objection
    Indefensible *(adjective)*
    Unsustainable *(adjective)*
    defective *(adjective)*
    Implausible *(adjective)*

Untoward *(adjective)*–Unexpected and inconvenient
    Inappropriate *(adjective)*
    Unanticipated *(adjective)*
    Unforeseen *(adjective)*
    Unpredictable *(adjective)*

Unsated *(adjective)*–Not having been satisfied
    Disappointed *(adjective)*
    Displeased *(adjective)*
    Unappeased *(adjective)*
    Unassuaged *(adjective)*

Upstart *(noun)*–A person who has risen suddenly in rank or importance
    Parvenue *(noun)*
    Social climber *(noun)*
    Name-dropper *(noun)*
    Nouveau riche *(noun)*

Upswing *(noun)*–An upward trend; an increase in strength or quantity
    Upturn *(noun)*
    Boom *(noun)*
    Growth *(noun)*
    Increase *(noun)*

Urn *(noun)*–A tall, rounded vase with a stem and base, especially one used for storing the ashes of a cremated person
    Jar *(noun)*
    Pitcher *(noun)*
    Ossuary *(noun)*
    Samovar *(noun)*

Usher *(noun)*–A person who shows people to their seats, especially in a cinema or theatre or at a wedding
    Attendant *(noun)*
    Escort *(noun)*
    Guide *(noun)*
    Aide *(noun)*

Usage *(noun)*–The action of using

V

something or the fact of being used
Employment *(noun)*
Consumption *(noun)*
Habit *(noun)*
Custom *(noun)*

Usurp *(verb)* –Take a position of power or importance illegally or by force
Seize *(verb)*
Appropriate *(verb)*
Wrest *(verb)*
Commandeer *(verb)*

Utopian *(adjective)*–Modelled on or aiming for a state in which everything is perfect
Idealistic *(adjective)*
Idyllic *(adjective)*
Elysian *(adjective)*
Perfect *(adjective)*

Vacant *(adjective)*–Empty; unoccupied
Deserted *(adjective)*
Unfilled *(adjective)*
Uninhabited *(adjective)*
Unused *(adjective)*

Vanish *(verb)* –Disappear
Dissolve *(verb)*
Evaporate *(verb)*
Fade *(verb)*
dematerialise *(verb)*

Victory *(noun)*–Win, success
Achievement *(noun)*

Triumph *(noun)*
Winning *(noun)*
Conquest *(noun)*

Virtue *(noun)*–Honour, integrity
Ethic *(noun)*
Goodness *(noun)*
Ideal *(noun)*
Morality *(noun)*

Visible *(adjective)*–Apparent, seeable
Conspicuous *(adjective)*
Detectable *(adjective)*
Discernible *(adjective)*
Noticeable *(adjective)*

Voluntary *(adjective)*–Willing
Independent *(adjective)*
Volunteer *(adjective)*
Chosen *(adjective)*
Free *(adjective)*

Vagary *(noun)*–An unexpected and inexplicable change in a situation or in someone's behaviour
Quirk *(noun)*
Idiosyncracy *(noun)*
Eccentricity *(noun)*
Whim *(noun)*

Vagabond *(noun)*–A person who wanders from place to place without a home or job
Wanderer *(noun)*

Nomad *(noun)*
Wayfarer *(noun)*
Gypsy *(noun)*

Vainglorious *(adjective)*–Someone who feels self-important
Arrogant *(adjective)*
Bragging *(adjective)*
Conceited *(adjective)*
Pompous *(adjective)*

Valet *(noun)*–A man's personal male attendant, who is responsible for his clothes and appearance
Attendant *(noun)*
Squire *(noun)*
Manservant *(noun)*
Dresser *(noun)*

Valetudinarian *(noun)*–A person who is unduly anxious about their health
Hypochondriac *(noun)*
Neurotic *(noun)*
Invalid *(noun)*
Morbid *(noun)*

Variegated *(adjective)*–Exhibiting different colours, especially as irregular patches or streaks
Checkered *(adjective)*
Motley *(adjective)*
Spotted *(adjective)*
Mottled *(adjective)*

Valise *(noun)*–A small travelling bag or suitcase
Baggage *(noun)*
Satchel *(noun)*
Haversack *(noun)*
Gripsack *(noun)*

Vane *(noun)*–A broad blade attached to a rotating axis which is pushed by wind or water
Feather *(noun)*
Fan *(noun)*
Weathercock *(noun)*

Vanguard *(noun)*–A group of people leading the way in new developments or ideas
Front *(noun)*
Pioneer *(noun)*
Lead *(noun)*
Radical *(noun)*

Vanquish *(verb)* –Defeat thoroughly
Conquer *(verb)*
trounce *(verb)*
Annihilate *(verb)*
Subjugate *(verb)*

Vaunt *(verb)* –Boast about or praise something excessively
Brag *(verb)*
Flaunt *(verb)*
Show off *(verb)*
Boast *(verb)*

Vaudeville *(noun)*–A type of entertainment popular chiefly in the US in the early 20th century, featuring burlesque comedy and song and dance
Theater *(noun)*
Skit *(noun)*
Show *(noun)*
Revue *(noun)*

Veer *(verb)* –Change direction suddenly
Swerve *(verb)*
career *(verb)*
Weave *(verb)*
Swing *(verb)*

Vehemence *(noun)*–Great forceful-ness or intensity of feeling or ex-pression
  Passion *(noun)*
  Ardour *(noun)*
  Fervour *(noun)*
  Urgency *(noun)*

Vellum *(noun)*–Fine parchment made originally from the skin of a calf
  Sheet *(noun)*
  Note *(noun)*
  Papyrus *(noun)*
  Pad *(noun)*

Veracity *(noun)*–Conformity to facts
  Accuracy *(noun)*
  Precision *(noun)*
  Realism *(noun)*
  Authenticity *(noun)*

Veritable *(adjective)*–Used for em-phasis, often to qualify a metaphor
  Actual *(adjective)*
  Factual *(adjective)*
  Genuine *(adjective)*
  legit *(adjective)*

Verdure *(noun)*–Lush green veg-etation
  Freshness *(adjective)*
  Greenery *(noun)*
  Frondescence *(noun)*
  Leafage *(noun)*

Versicolor *(adjective)*–Multicolour
  Kaleidoscope *(adjective)*
  Polychromatic *(adjective)*
  Varicolored *(adjective)*
  Variegated *(adjective)*

Verve *(noun)*–Vigour and spirit or enthusiasm

  Energy *(noun)*
  Vitality *(noun)*
  Vivacity *(noun)*
  Animation *(noun)*

Vial *(noun)*–A small container, used especially for holding liquid medicines
  Bottle *(noun)*
  Phial *(noun)*
  Ampoule *(noun)*
  Flask *(noun)*

Vicar *(noun)*–An incumbent of a parish in the Church of England
  Pastor *(noun)*
  Clergyman *(noun)*
  Minister *(noun)*
  Priest *(noun)*

Victuals *(noun)*–Food or provisions
  Eatables *(noun)*
  Edibles *(noun)*
  Snacks *(noun)*
  Meal *(noun)*

Vie *(verb)* –Compete eagerly with someone in order to do or achieve something
  Contend *(verb)*
  Contest *(verb)*
  Fight *(verb)*
  Battle *(verb)*

Virulence *(noun)*–To resent some-thing or someone strongly
  Animosity *(noun)*
  Acrimony *(noun)*
  Grudge *(noun)*
  Embitterment *(noun)*

Virtuoso *(noun)*–A person highly skilled in music or another artistic pursuit

Genius *(noun)*
Expert *(noun)*
Maestro *(noun)*
Prodigy *(noun)*

Virtuosity *(noun)*–Great skill in music or another artistic pursuit
Mastery *(noun)*
Expertise *(noun)*
Prowess *(noun)*
Brilliance *(noun)*

Vicarious *(adjective)*–Experienced in the imagination through the feelings or actions of another person
Secondary *(adjective)*
Derivative *(adjective)*
Surrogate *(adjective)*
Substitute *(adjective)*

Vignette *(noun)*–A brief evocative description, account or episode
Scene *(noun)*
Sketch *(noun)*
Picture *(noun)*
Story *(noun)*

Vigil *(noun)*–A period of keeping awake during the time usually spent asleep, especially to keep watch or pray
Patrol *(noun)*
Lookout *(noun)*
Nightwatch *(noun)*
Surveillance *(noun)*

Virago *(noun)*–A domineering, violent or bad-tempered woman

Harridan *(noun)*
Shrew *(noun)*
Termagant *(noun)*
Vixen *(noun)*

Visage *(noun)*–A person's face, with reference to the form or proportions of the features
Countenance *(noun)*
Aspect *(noun)*
Features *(noun)*
Mien *(noun)*

Visceral *(adjective)*–Relating to deep inward feelings rather than to the intellect *(adjective)*
Innate *(adjective)*
Intuitive *(adjective)*
Intrinsic *(adjective)*

Vicissitude *(noun)*–A change of circumstances or fortune, typically one that is unwelcome or unpleasant
Alteration *(noun)*
Transformation *(noun)*
Metamorphosis *(noun)*
Transition *(noun)*

Vista *(noun)*–A pleasing view
Prospect *(noun)*
Panorama *(noun)*
Spectacle *(noun)*
Sight *(noun)*

Vociferous *(adjective)*–Expressing or characterised by vehement opin-

W

ions
Outspoken
Vocal *(adjective)*
Frank *(adjective)*
Candid *(adjective)*

Volition *(noun)*–The faculty or power of using one's will
Choice *(noun)*
Option *(noun)*
Willingness *(noun)*
Choosing *(noun)*

Votarist *(noun)*–Person overenthusiastic about interest
Afficionado *(noun)*
Fanatic *(noun)*
Addict *(noun)*
Enthusiast *(noun)*

Waft *(verb)* –Pass or cause to pass gently through the air
Drift *(verb)*
Float *(verb)*
Glide *(verb)*
Whirl *(verb)*

Waif *(noun)*–A homeless, neglected, or abandoned person, especially a child
Orphan *(noun)*
Stray *(noun)*
Outcast *(noun)*
Ragamuffin *(noun)*

Wallow *(verb)* –Indulge in an unrestrained way in something that one finds pleasurable
Luxuriate *(verb)*
Bask *(verb)*
Revel *(verb)*
Glory *(verb)*

Wan *(adjective)*–Pale and giving the impression of illness or exhaustion
Pallid *(adjective)*
Ashen *(adjective)*
White *(adjective)*
Grey *(adjective)*

Warble *(verb)* –Sing softly and with a succession of constantly changing notes
Trill *(verb)*
Chirp *(verb)*
Tweet *(verb)*
Peep *(verb)*

Warp *(verb)* –Make or become bent or twisted out of shape
Distort *(verb)*
Deform *(verb)*
Misshape *(verb)*
Contort *(verb)*

Wart *(noun)*–A small, hard, benign growth on the skin
Lump *(noun)*
Swelling *(noun)*
Protuberance *(noun)*

Corn *(noun)*

Wassail *(noun)*–Celebration
Bash *(noun)*
Frolic *(noun)*
Gala *(noun)*
Party *(noun)*

Washout *(noun)*–Failure
Disaster *(noun)*
Fiasco *(noun)*
Debacle *(noun)*
Flop *(noun)*

Waspish *(adjective)*–Readily expressing anger or irritation
Touchy *(adjective)*
Testy *(adjective)*
Irascible *(adjective)*
Moody *(adjective)*

Wayfarer *(noun)*–A person who travels on foot
Traveller *(noun)*
Nomad *(noun)*
Gypsy *(noun)*
Vagabond *(noun)*

Wastrel *(noun)*–A wasteful or good for nothing person
Spendthrift *(noun)*
Prodigal *(noun)*
Profligate *(noun)*
squanderer *(noun)*

Wellspring *(noun)*–An abundant source of something
Fountain *(noun)*
Fountainhead *(noun)*
Source *(noun)*
Origin *(noun)*

Weighty *(adjective)*–Weighing a great deal
Heavy *(adjective)*

Bulky *(adjective)*
Hefty *(adjective)*
Cumbersome *(adjective)*

Weak *(adjective)*–Not strong
Feeble *(adjective)*
Fragile *(adjective)*
Sickly *(adjective)*
Weakened *(adjective)*

Wet *(adjective)*–Damp, moist
Rainy *(adjective)*
Soaked *(adjective)*
Soggy *(adjective)*
Moistened *(adjective)*

Wide *(adjective)*–Expansive, roomy
Broad *(adjective)*
Expanded *(adjective)*
Spacious *(adjective)*
Vast *(adjective)*

Win *(noun)*–Victory
Accomplishment *(noun)*
Achievement *(noun)*
Success *(noun)*
Triumph *(noun)*

Wisdom *(noun)*–Insight, common sense
Foresight *(noun)*
Knowledge *(noun)*
Savvy *(noun)*
Understanding *(noun)*

Wrong *(adjective)*–Incorrect
Erroneous *(adjective)*
False *(adjective)*
Inaccurate *(adjective)*
Unsound *(adjective)*

Wean *(verb)* –Accustom to food other than its mother's milk
Discourage *(verb)*

Halt *(verb)*
Remove *(verb)*
Unaccustom *(verb)*

Weasel *(noun)*–A deceitful or treacherous person
Scoundrel *(noun)*
Wretch *(noun)*
Rogue *(noun)*
Knave *(noun)*

Wharf *(noun)*–A level quayside area to which a ship may be moored to load and unload
Quay *(noun)*
Pier *(noun)*
Berth *(noun)*
Jetty *(noun)*

Wheedle *(verb)* –Use endearments or flattery to persuade someone to do something or give one something
Coax *(verb)*
Cajole *(verb)*
Beguile *(verb)*
Influence *(verb)*

Wherewithal *(noun)*–The money or other means needed for a particular purpose
Money *(noun)*

cash *(noun)*
capital *(noun)*
Finances *(noun)*

Whirligig *(verb)* –Revolve
Twirl *(verb)*
Whirl *(verb)*
Spin *(verb)*
Spiral *(verb)*

Wisecrack *(noun)*–A witty remark or joke
Witticism *(noun)*
Quip *(noun)*
Jest *(noun)*
Sally *(noun)*

Withal *(adverb)* –In addition to
Besides *(adverb)*
Additionally *(adverb)*
Conjointly *(adverb)*
Together with *(adverb)*

Wraith *(noun)*–A ghost or ghost-like image of someone, especially one seen shortly before or after their death
Spectre *(noun)*
Phantom *(noun)*
Spirit *(noun)*
Apparition *(noun)*

Wreck *(verb)* –Destroy or severely damage

Y

Demolish *(verb)*
Ruin *(verb)*
Vandalise *(verb)*
Smash *(verb)*

Wretch *(noun)*–An unfortunate person
Miserable *(adjective)*
Sad *(adjective)*
poor *(adjective)*
Unhappy *(adjective)*

Writhe *(verb)* –Make twisting, squirming movements or contortions of the body
Wriggle *(verb)*
Thrash *(verb)*
Flail *(verb)*
Twitch *(verb)*

Yacht *(noun)*–A medium-sized sailing boat equipped for cruising or racing
Sailboat *(noun)*
Cruiser *(noun)*
Racer *(noun)*
Sloop *(noun)*

Yammer *(verb)* –Make a loud, repetitive noise
Howl *(verb)*
Yowl *(verb)*
Carp *(verb)*
Wail *(verb)*

Yaw *(verb)* –Swerve

Curve *(verb)*
deviate *(verb)*
Veer *(verb)*
Weave *(verb)*

Yodel *(verb)* –Sing
Carol *(verb)*
Shout *(verb)*
Trill *(verb)*
Warble *(verb)*

Yank *(verb)* –Pull with a jerk
Tug *(verb)*
Wrench *(verb)*
Pluck *(verb)*
Snatch *(verb)*

Yardstick *(noun)*–A measuring rod a yard long, typically divided into inches
Barometer *(noun)*
benchmark *(noun)*
Guideline *(noun)*
Standard *(noun)*

Yearling *(noun)*–An animal, especially a sheep, calf, or foal that is a year old
Nursling *(noun)*
Weanling *(noun)*
Young bull *(noun)*
Young cow *(noun)*

Yeoman *(noun)*–Worker
Assistant *(noun)*
Attendant *(noun)*

Z

Servant *(noun)*
Subordinate *(noun)*

Yoke *(noun)*–A wooden crosspiece that is fastened over the necks of two animals and attached to the plough or cart that they are to pull
Harness *(noun)*
Collar *(noun)*
Tackle *(noun)*
Tack *(noun)*

Young *(adjective)*–Immature
Budding *(adjective)*
Inexperienced *(adjective)*
New *(adjective)*
Youthful *(adjective)*

Zany *(adjective)*–Amusingly unconventional and idiosyncratic
Odd *(adjective)*
Quirky *(adjective)*
Ludicrous *(adjective)*
Peculiar *(adjective)*

Zealot *(noun)*–A person who is fanatical and uncompromising in pursuit of their religious, political or other ideals
Extremist *(noun)*
Radical *(noun)*
Fanatic *(noun)*
Militant *(noun)*

Zenith *(noun)*–The time at which

ANTONYMS

ANTONYMS

The word, 'antonym' was coined in the 19th century by the philogogists. The word, antonym comes from the Greek word, *anti (opposite)* and *onoma (name)*. This suggests that antonyms are words which have opposite meanings. The term, 'antonym' is synonymous with opposite. Antonyms tend to be *adverbs, adjectives* and *verbs* with relatively few nouns. Words opposite to each other may be similar in most other respects. One word may have more than one antonym.

Generally, our day to day English Vocabulary consists of antonyms and in order to improve ones' vocabulary one needs to be familiar with them as they play an important role in helping to build a strong base of English.

For example:

An antonym for 'behave' would be 'misbehave'. Similarly, the opposite or antonym for 'agree' would be 'disagree'.

Inside –Outside

Balance –Imbalance

Dependent –Independent, etc.

A

About	:	Exactly	**Accord**	:	Disagreement
Above	:	Below	**Accost**	:	Ignore
Abundance	:	Lack	**Adjudge**	:	Defer
To accept	:	To refuse	**Acquit**	:	Accuse
Accidental	:	Intentional	**Adjust**	:	Disarrange
Compulsory	:	Optional	**Adjoin**	:	Disconnect
Active	:	Lazy	**Avouch**	:	Abandon
To add	:	To subtract	**Aplomb**	:	Fear
To admit	:	To deny	**Accept**	:	Fail
Adapt	:	Neglect	**Affirm**	:	Deny
Adept	:	Incapable	**Abduct**	:	Release
Astute	:	Foolish	**Acumen**	:	Ignorance
Abase	:	Honour	**Aching**	:	Healthy
Abhor	:	Admire	**Amaze**	:	Bore
Abject	:	Commendable	**Apex**	:	Base
Abduct	:	Release	**Advice**	:	Opposition
Abomination	:	Delight	**Abysmal**	:	Low
Ablaze	:	Dim	**Astound**	:	Clarify
Abrasive	:	Mild	**Affect**	:	Dissuade
Abstain	:	Indulge	**Abase**	:	Grow
Abstract	:	Real	**Abhor**	:	Admire
Asinine	:	Meaningful	**Adult**	:	Child
Assure	:	Dissuade	**Advanced**	:	Elementary
Abject	:	Commendable	**Affirmative**	:	Negative
Adjourn	:	Advance	**Afraid**	:	Brave

After → All

After	:	Before
Against	:	For
Alike	:	Different
Alive	:	Dead
All	:	None
Always	:	Never
Ancient	:	Modern
To agree	:	To refuse, to argue
To allow	:	To forbid
Already	:	Not yet
Always	:	Never
Amateur	:	Professional
Ambivalent	:	Determined
Amiable	:	Hostile
Amicable	:	Disagreeable
Ample	:	Cramped
Animosity	:	Humane
Annihilate	:	Establish
Anomaly	:	Conformity
Anonymous	:	Identified
Anticipate	:	Doubt
Antipathy	:	Friendship
Apathy	:	Concern
Aptitude	:	Dislike
Arbitrary	:	Consistent
Arcane	:	Well:Known
Archaic	:	Contemporary
Archetype	:	Atypical
Ardent	:	Apathetic
Arduous	:	Easy
Aristocratic	:	Poor

Artifice	:	Honesty
Ascetic	:	Social
To amuse	:	To bore
Angel	:	Devil
Animosity	:	Humane
To annoy	:	To satisfy
To answer	:	To ask
Answer	:	Question
Apart	:	Together
Approximately	:	Exactly
To argue	:	To agree
To arrest	:	To free, to set free
Arrival	:	Departure
Artificial	:	Natural
Asleep	:	Awake
Attack	:	Defence, protection
Attic	:	Cellar
Awful	:	Delicious, nice, pleasant
Absent	:	Present
Abundant	:	Scarce
Accept	:	Decline, refuse
Accurate	:	Inaccurate
Admire	:	Despise
Admit	:	Deny
Advantage	:	Disadvantage
Against	:	For
Agree	:	Disagree
Alive	:	Dead
All	:	None, nothing

Ally → Awake

Ally	:	Enemy	**Arrive**	:	Depart
Ancient	:	Modern	**Artificial**	:	Natural
Antonym	:	Synonym	**Ascend**	:	Descend
Apart	:	Together	**Attic**	:	Cellar
Appear	:	Disappear, vanish	**Attractive**	:	Repulsive
Approve	:	Disapprove	**Awake**	:	Asleep

B

Back	:	Front
Background	:	Foreground
Backward	:	Forward
Bad	:	Good
Bad luck	:	Good luck
Baffle	:	Explain
Baleful	:	Auspicious
Balk	:	Accept
Ban	:	Approval
Banish	:	Allow
Barbaric	:	Civilised
Barrage	:	Dribble
Barren	:	Fruitful
Bastion	:	Weakness
Befuddle	:	Enlighten
Beguile	:	Refuse
Behemoth	:	Lightweight
Beholden	:	Ungrateful
Behoove	:	Unsuitable
Belittle	:	Approve
Belligerent	:	Agreeable
Bemoan	:	Praise
Bemused	:	Disinterested
Benign	:	Unfriendly
Benevolent	:	Cruel

Berate	:	Compliment
Beseech	:	Command, answer
Besmirch	:	Clean, praise, honour
Bestow	:	Deny
Bias	:	Fairness
Bicker	:	Agree
Bifurcate	:	Join
Bilateral	:	Multilateral
Billowing	:	Shrink
Binge	:	Saving
Bland	:	Exciting
Beauty	:	Ugliness
Before	:	After
To begin	:	To end, to finish
Beginning	:	Ending
Behind	:	In front of
Blunt	:	Sharp
Body	:	Soul
To bore	:	To amuse, to be interested in
Boring	:	Interesting, exciting
To borrow	:	To lend

Bottom → Broad

Bottom	:	Top		
Boy	:	Girl		
Brave	:	Timid, cowardly		
To break	:	To mend, to fix		
Broad	:	Narrow		
Brother	:	Sister		
To build	:	To destroy		
Busy	:	Lazy		
To buy	:	To sell		
Backward	:	Forward		
Bad	:	Good		
Beautiful	:	Ugly		
Before	:	After		
Begin	:	End		
Below	:	Above		
Bent	:	Straight		
Best	:	Worst		
Better	:	Worse		

Big	:	Little, small
Birth	:	Death
Black	:	White
Blame	:	Praise
Bless	:	Curse
Blare	:	Toot
Blasphemy	:	Respect
Bleak	:	Bright
Blatant	:	Concealed
Blunt	:	Sharp
Bitter	:	Sweet
Bold	:	Meek, timid
Borrow	:	Lend
Bound	:	Unbound, free
Boundless	:	Limited
Bright	:	Dim, dull
Brighten	:	Fade
Broad	:	Narrow

C

Cacophonous	:	Quiet	Ceiling	:	Floor
Calamity	:	Creation	Cellar	:	Attic
Callow	:	Experienced	Centre	:	Periphery, outskirts, suburb
Candid	:	Biased			
Capitulate	:	Conquer	Certainly	:	Probably
Capricious	:	Cautious	Changeable	:	Constant
Castigate	:	Approve	Cheap	:	Expensive
Caustic	:	Bland	Child	:	Adult, grown up
Cease	:	Begin			
Cede	:	Fight	Children	:	Parents
Chagrin	:	Confidence	Clean	:	Dirty
Challenge	:	Acceptance	Clever	:	Stupid
Charisma	:	Dull	To close	:	To open
Chastise	:	Laud	Closed	:	Opened/Open
Chronic	:	Halting	Cloudy	:	Clear, sunny, bright
Circumspect	:	Careless			
Clandestine	:	Forthright	Can	:	Cannot, can't
Clemency	:	Meanness	Capable	:	Incapable
Clique	:	Individual	Captive	:	Free
Coercion	:	Consent	Careful	:	Careless
Calm	:	Windy, troubled	Cheap	:	Expensive
			Cheerful	:	Sad, discouraged, dreary
Calm	:	Excited			
Careful	:	Careless	Clear	:	Cloudy, opaque
To catch	:	To miss, to throw			

Clever	:	Stupid	**Courage**	:	Fear
Clockwise	:	Counterclockwise anticlockwis'e	**Courageous**	:	Cowardly
			To create	:	To destroy
Close	:	Far, distant	**Cruel**	:	Kind, humane
Clumsy	:	Graceful	**To cry**	:	To laugh
Cold	:	Hot	**Curly**	:	Straight
Cold (noun)	:	Heat	**Combine**	:	Separate
To come	:	To go	**Come**	:	Go
Comedy	:	Tragedy	**Comfort**	:	Discomfort
Complicated	:	Simple	**Common**	:	Rare
Compliment	:	Insult	**Conceal**	:	Reveal
Compulsory	:	Voluntary	**Contract**	:	Expand
To connect	:	To separate	**Cool**	:	Warm
Consonant	:	Vowel	**Correct**	:	Incorrect, wrong
Constant	:	Variable, changeable			
Construction	:	Destruction	**Courage**	:	Cowardice
To continue	:	To interrupt	**Create**	:	Destroy
Cool	:	Warm	**Crooked**	:	Straight
Correct	:	False, wrong	**Compulsory**	:	Voluntary
			Courteous	:	Discourteous, rude

D

To damage	:	To repair	**Diabolical**	:	Good
Delay	:	Hasten	**Diatribe**	:	Praise
Dapper	:	Scruffy	**Dichotomy**	:	Similarity
Dauntless	:	Afraid	**Diffident**	:	Confident
Dawdle	:	Hurry	**Dilettante or Novice**	:	Professional
Dearth	:	Abundance			
Debacle	:	Accomplishment	**Dire**	:	Unimportant, trivial
Debilitate	:	Strengthen			
Debunk	:	Prove	**Danger**	:	Security, safety
Deduce	:	Reject			
Defame	:	Praise	**Dangerous**	:	Safe
Defiance	:	Submission	**Dark**	:	Light
Defunct	:	Existing	**Daughter**	:	Son
Dejected	:	Encouraged	**Dawn**	:	Dusk
Deluge	:	Drizzle	**Day**	:	Night
Denounce	:	Applaud	**Deep**	:	Shallow
Depict	:	Hide	**Defeat**	:	Victory
Deplete	:	Fill	**Delicious**	:	Tasteless, awful
Derivation	:	Conclusion			
Desolate	:	Inhabited	**To deny**	:	To admit
Destitute	:	Solvent	**To depart**	:	To arrive
Deter	:	Assist	**Departure**	:	Arrival
Detrimental	:	Beneficial	**Desperate**	:	Hopeful
Devout	:	Apathetic	**Devil**	:	Angel
Dexterity	:	Clumsiness	**Dictatorship**	:	Democracy
			To die	:	To live

Dirty → Dreary

Dirty	:	Clean	**Day**	:	Night
Disease	:	Healthy	**Daytime**	:	Night-time
Distant	:	Near	**Dead**	:	Alive
Division	:	Unity	**Decline**	:	Accept
To divorce	:	To marry	**Decrease**	:	Increase
Divorce	:	Marriage	**Deep**	:	Shallow
Divorced	:	Married	**Definite**	:	Indefinite
Domestic	:	Foreign	**Demand**	:	Supply
Down	:	Up	**Despair**	:	Hope
Downstairs	:	Upstairs	**Dim**	:	Bright
Dry	:	Humid or wet	**Disappear**	:	Appear
Dull	:	Interesting	**Discourage**	:	Encourage
Dusk	:	Dawn	**Downwards**	:	Upwards
Dangerous	:	Safe	**Dreary**	:	Cheerful
Dark	:	Light			

E

Early	:	Late	**Exposure**	:	Shelter
East	:	West	**Extreme**	:	Moderate
Easy	:	Difficult, hard	**East**	:	West
Elementary	:	Advanced	**Elegant**	:	Crude, inelegant
To emigrate	:	To immigrate			
Emigration	:	Immigration	**Elementary**	:	Advanced
Empty	:	Full	**Empty**	:	Full
To end	:	To begin	**Encourage**	:	Discourage
Beginning	:	Ending	**End**	:	Begin, start
Enemy	:	Friend	**Ending**	:	Beginning
To enjoy	:	To detest	**Enemy**	:	Friend
To enter	:	To leave	**Enigma**	:	Simple
Entrance	:	Exit	**Eager**	:	Disinterested
Equal	:	Different	**Emphatic**	:	Vague
Even	:	Odd	**Embellish**	:	Simplify
Evening	:	Morning	**Endearing**	:	Offensive
Everybody	:	Nobody	**Envelope**	:	Interior
Everything	:	Nothing	**Entice**	:	Repel
Exactly	:	Approximately	**Enduring**	:	Obsolete
Excited	:	Calm	**Engage**	:	Retreat
Exciting	:	Boring	**Entrap**	:	Free
To exclude	:	To include	**Enjoy**	:	Hate
Exit	:	Entrance	**Enter**	:	Exit
Expensive	:	Cheap	**Entrance**	:	Exit
Export	:	Import	**Equal**	:	Different

Even → External

Even	:	Odd	**Exciting**	:	Boring
Evening	:	Morning	**Expand**	:	Contract
Everybody	:	Nobody	**Export**	:	Import
Everything	:	Nothing	**Exterior**	:	Interior
Exactly	:	Approximately	**External**	:	Internal
Excited	:	Calm			

F

Fade	:	Brighten	To form	:	To destroy
Fail	:	Succeed	Fortune	:	Bad luck
False	:	True	Forward	:	Backward
Famous	:	Unknown	To free	:	To arrest
Famished	:	Satisfied	To freeze	:	To melt
Far	:	Near	Frequently	:	Occasionally
Fascinate	:	Displease	Friend	:	Enemy
Fasten	:	Sever	Front	:	Rear
Faith	:	Distrust	In front of	:	Back, behind
Fast	:	Slow	Full	:	Empty
Fat	:	Thin	Funny	:	Serious
Feeble	:	Strong, powerful	Future	:	Past, present
Few	:	Many	Find	:	Lose
Finish	:	Start	First	:	Last
First	:	Final, last	Float	:	Sink
To fix	:	To break	Foolish	:	Wise
Flat	:	Hilly	Fore	:	Aft
Floor	:	Ceiling	Free	:	Bound, captive
To follow	:	To lead	Fold	:	Unfold
To forbid	:	To allow, to let, to permit	Forget	:	Remember
			Found	:	Lost
For	:	Against	Fresh	:	Stale
Foreground	:	Background	Frequent	:	Seldom
Foreign	:	Domestic	Friend	:	Enemy
Foreigner	:	Native	For	:	Against
To forget	:	To remember	Fortunate	:	Unfortunate
			Full	:	Empty

G

General	:	Particular, special	**Gentle**	:	Rough
Generous	:	Mean	**Get**	:	Give
Gentle	:	Violent, rough, strict	**Giant**	:	Tiny, small, dwarf
Gentleman	:	Lady	**Girl**	:	Boy
Girl	:	Boy	**Give**	:	Receive, take
To give	:	To take	**Glad**	:	Sad, sorry
To go	:	To come, to stop	**Gloomy**	:	Cheerful
Good	:	Bad	**Go**	:	Stop
Godfather	:	Godmother	**Good**	:	Bad, evil
Grown Up	:	Child	**Grant**	:	Refuse
Guest	:	Host	**Great**	:	Tiny, small, unimportant
Guilty	:	Innocent	**Grow**	:	Shrink
Generous	:	Stingy	**Guest**	:	Host
			Guilty	:	Innocent

H

Happy	:	Sad		**Host**	:	Guest, visitor
Happiness	:	Sadness		**Hot**	:	Cold
Happy	:	Sad		**Huge**	:	Tiny
Handsome	:	Ugly		**Human**	:	Animal
Hard	:	Easy, soft		**Humane**	:	Cruel
To hate	:	To enjoy, to like, to love		**Humid**	:	Dry
				Hungry	:	Thirsty
To harvest	:	To plant		**Husband**	:	Wife
Hasten	:	Slow down		**Hard**	:	Easy
Hasty	:	Unhurried		**Hard**	:	Soft
Haughty	:	Modest		**Harmful**	:	Harmless
Health	:	Disease, illness		**Harsh**	:	Mild
Healthy	:	Ill, sick		**Hate**	:	Love
Heave	:	Drop		**Haves**	:	Have-nots
Heaven	:	Hell		**Healthy**	:	Diseased, ill sick
Heavy	:	Light				
Hell	:	Heaven		**Heaven**	:	Hell
Here	:	There		**Heavy**	:	Light
High	:	Deep		**Help**	:	Hinder
High	:	Low		**Here**	:	There
Hilly	:	Flat		**Hero**	:	Coward
To hit	:	To miss		**High**	:	Low
Hopeful	:	Desperate, hopeless		**Hill**	:	Valley
				Hinder	:	Help
Hopeless	:	Hopeful		**Honest**	:	Dishonest
Horizontal	:	Vertical		**Hopeful**	:	Hopeless

117

Horizontal → Husband

Horizontal	:	Vertical	**Humane**	:	Cruel
Hot	:	Cold	**Humble**	:	Proud
Host	:	Guest	**Humid**	:	Dry
Huge	:	Tiny	**Hungry**	:	Satisfied, full
Human	:	Animal	**Husband**	:	Wife

I

Ignore	:	Notices
To Ignore	:	To notice
Ill	:	Healthy, well
Immense	:	Tiny, small
Immigrate	:	Emigrate
To immigrate	:	To emigrate
Important	:	Trivial
Immigration	:	Emigration
Import	:	Export
In	:	Out
Include	:	Exclude
To include	:	To exclude
Inconstancy	:	Steadfastness
Increase	:	Decrease
To increase	:	To reduce
Inferior	:	Superior
Innocent	:	Guilty
Inhale	:	Exhale

Ingenious	:	Uninspired
Inner	:	Outer
Innocent	:	Guilty
Inside	:	Outside
Insult	:	Compliment
Intentional	:	Accidental
Interested	:	Bored
Interesting	:	Boring, dull
To interrupt	:	To continue
Intelligent	:	Stupid, unintelligent
Interesting	:	Boring
Interior	:	Exterior
Interesting	:	Dull, uninteresting
Internal	:	External
Intentional	:	Accidental
To jeopardise	:	To secure

J,K

Join	:	Separate		**Kind**	:	Cruel, nasty
Junior	:	Senior		**Knowledge**	:	Ignorance
Just	:	Unjust		**Known**	:	Unknown
Justice	:	Injustice				

L

Lack	:	Abundance, plenty
Lady	:	Gentleman
To land	:	To take off
Land	:	Water
Large	:	Small
Last	:	First
Late	:	Early
To laugh	:	To cry
Lazy	:	Active, busy
To lead	:	To follow
To learn	:	To teach
To leave	:	To arrive, to enter
Left	:	Right
To lend	:	To borrow
Less	:	More
To let	:	To forbid
To lie	:	To stand
Life	:	Death
Light	:	Dark, heavy
To like	:	To hate
Liquid	:	Solid
Little	:	Big, large
Little	:	Much
To live	:	To die
Long	:	Short
To lose	:	To find, to win
Loser	:	Winner
Loud	:	Quiet
To love	:	To hate
Lovely	:	Terrible
Low	:	High
To lower	:	To raise
Landlord	:	Tenant
Large	:	Small
Last	:	First
Laugh	:	Cry
Lawful	:	Unlawful, illegal
Lazy	:	Industrious
Leader	:	Follower
Learn	:	Teach
Leave	:	Arrive
Let	:	Forbid
Left	:	Right
Lend	:	Borrow
Lengthen	:	Shorten
Lenient	:	Strict
Left	:	Right
Less	:	More
Life	:	Death

Light → Loyal

Light	:	Dark, heavy	**Lose**	:	Find
Like	:	Dislike, hate	**Loss**	:	Win
Likely	:	Unlikely	**Loud**	:	Quiet
Limited	:	Boundless	**Love**	:	Hate
Little	:	Big	**Low**	:	High
Long	:	Short	**Loyal**	:	Disloyal
Loose	:	Tight			

M

Mad	:	Happy, sane	**Moderate**	:	Extreme
Major	:	Minor	**Modern**	:	Ancient, old
Male	:	Female	**Monarchy**	:	Republic
Man	:	Woman	**Moon**	:	Sun
Many	:	Few, some	**More**	:	Less
Marriage	:	Divorce	**Morning**	:	Evening
Married	:	Divorced,	**Mountain**	:	Valley
		single	**Much**	:	Little
To marry	:	To divorce	**Malicious**	:	Benevolent
Master	:	Servant	**Many**	:	Few
Maximum	:	Minimum	**Mature**	:	Immature
Mean	:	Generous	**Maximum**	:	Minimum
To melt	:	To freeze	**Melt**	:	Freeze
Men	:	Women	**Merry**	:	Sad
To mend	:	To break	**Messy**	:	Neat
Mess	:	Order	**Minor**	:	Major
Midnight	:	Noon	**Minority**	:	Majority
Minimum	:	Maximum	**Miser**	:	Spendthrift
Minor	:	Major	**Misunderstand**	:	Understand
To miss	:	To hit, to catch	**More**	:	Less

N

Nadir	:	Zenith
Narrow	:	Broad, wide
Nasty	:	Nice, pleasant
Native	:	Foreigner, stranger
Natural	:	Artificial
Near	:	Distant, far
Negative	:	Affirmative
Nephew	:	Niece
Never	:	Always
New	:	Ancient, old
Nice	:	Awful, nasty
Niece	:	Nephew
Night	:	Day
No	:	Yes
Nobody	:	Everybody
Noisy	:	Quiet, silent
Noon	:	Midnight

None of	:	All of
Normal	:	Strange
North	:	South
Not yet	:	Already
Nothing	:	Everything
To notice	:	To ignore
Now	:	Then
Near	:	Far, distant
Neat	:	Messy, untidy
Never	:	Always
New	:	Old
Night	:	Day
Night time	:	Daytime
No	:	Yes
Noisy	:	Quiet
None	:	Some
North	:	South

O

Occasionally	:	Frequently	**Order**	:	Mess
Occupied	:	Vacant	**Ordinary**	:	Special
Odd	:	Even	**Other**	:	Same
Off	:	On	**Out**	:	In
Often	:	Seldom, sometimes	**Obedient**	:	Disobedient
Offer	:	Refuse	**Old**	:	Young
Old	:	Modern, new, young	**Old**	:	New
			On	:	Off
On	:	Off	**Open**	:	Closed, shut
To open	:	To close, to shut	**Opposite**	:	Same, similar
			Optimist	:	Pessimist
Open	:	Closed, shut	**Out**	:	In
Opponent	:	Supporter	**Outer**	:	Inner
			Over	:	Under

P

Parents	:	Children		**Protection**	:	Attack
Part	:	Whole		**Public**	:	Private
Partial	:	Total		**To pull**	:	To push
Particular	:	General		**Pupil**	:	Teacher
To pass	:	To fail		**To push**	:	To pull
Past	:	Future, present		**Past**	:	Present
Peace	:	War		**Patient**	:	Impatient
To permit	:	To forbid		**Peace**	:	War
To plant	:	To harvest		**Permanent**	:	Temporary
Plenty	:	Lack		**Plentiful**	:	Scarce
Pleasant	:	Awful		**Plural**	:	Singular
Polite	:	Rude, impolite		**Poetry**	:	Prose
Poor	:	Rich, wealthy		**Polite**	:	Rude, impolite
Poverty	:	Wealth		**Possible**	:	Impossible
Powerful	:	Weak		**Poverty**	:	Wealth, riches
Presence	:	Absence		**Powerful**	:	Weak
Present	:	Past, future		**Pretty**	:	Ugly
Pretty	:	Ugly		**Private**	:	Public
Private	:	Public		**Prudent**	:	Imprudent
Probably	:	Certainly		**Pure**	:	Impure, contaminated
Professional	:	Amateur		**Push**	:	Pull
To protect	:	To attack				

Q,R

Qualified	:	Unqualified
Question	:	Answer
Quiet	:	Loud, noisy
Raise	:	Lower
Rapid	:	Slow
Rare	:	Common
To raise	:	To lower
Rainy	:	Sunny
Rear	:	Front
To receive	:	To send
To reduce	:	To increase
To refuse	:	To agree, to accept
Regret	:	Satisfaction
To remember	:	To forget
To repair	:	To damage
To reply	:	To ask
Reply	:	Question
Republic	:	Dictatorship, monarchy
To rest	:	To work
Rich	:	Poor
Right	:	Left, wrong

To rise	:	To sink
Rough	:	Gentle, smooth, soft
Rude	:	Polite
Rural	:	Urban
To take	:	To give
Loser	:	Winner
Loud	:	Quiet
To love	:	To hate
Lovely	:	Terrible
Low	:	High
To lower	:	To raise
There	:	Here
Then	:	Now
Thin	:	Thick, fat
To raise	:	To lower
Sunny	:	Tight
To receive	:	To send
To divorce	:	To marry
To refuse	:	To agree, to accept
Regret	:	Satisfaction
To remember	:	To forget

To reply → Rude

To reply	:	To ask	**Rich**	:	Poor
Regular	:	Irregular	**Right**	:	Left, wrong
Real	:	Fake	**Rough**	:	Smooth
			Rude	:	Courteous

S

Safe	:	Unsafe	**Sober**	:	Drunk
Same	:	Opposite	**Soft**	:	Hard
Satisfactory	:	Unsatisfactory	**Some**	:	None
Secure	:	Insecure	**Sorrow**	:	Joy
Scatter	:	Collect	**Sour**	:	Sweet
Separate	:	Join, together	**Sow**	:	reap
Serious	:	Trivial	**Straight**	:	Crooked
Second	:	Hand-New	**Start**	:	Finish
Shallow	:	Deep	**Stop**	:	Go
Shrink	:	Grow	**Strict**	:	Lenient
Sick	:	Healthy, ill	**Strong**	:	Weak
Simple	:	Complex, hard	**Success**	:	Failure
Singular	:	Plural	**Sunny**	:	Cloudy
Sink	:	Float	**Synonym**	:	Antonym
Slim	:	Fat, thick	**Sweet**	:	Sour
Slow	:	Fast	**Sweltering**	:	Freezing

T

Take	:	Give		**Together**	:	Apart
Tall	:	Short		**Top**	:	Bottom
Tame	:	Wild		**Tough**	:	Easy, tender
Them	:	Us		**Transparent**	:	Opaque
There	:	Here		**True**	:	False
Thick	:	Thin		**Truth**	:	Falsehood, lie, untruth
Tight	:	Loose, slack		**To trust**	:	To suspect
Tiny	:	Big, huge				

U

Ugliness	:	Beauty	**Up**	:	Down
Ugly	:	Beautiful, handsome, pretty	**Upside-Down**	:	Right-side-Up
Under	:	Over	**Upstairs**	:	Downstairs
To unite	:	To divide, to separate	**Urban**	:	Rural
			Upstairs	:	Downstairs
Unfold	:	Fold	**Urgent**	:	Leisurely
Unity	:	Division	**Useless**	:	Useful
Unknown	:	Known	**Us**	:	Them
Unqualified	:	Qualified	**Useful**	:	Useless
Unsafe	:	Safe			

V

Vacant	:	Occupied	**Vowel**	:	Consonant
Valley	:	Mountain	**Vacant**	:	Occupied
Vertical	:	Horizontal	**Vanish**	:	Appear
Victory	:	Defeat	**Vast**	:	Tiny
To whisper	:	To shout, scream	**Victory**	:	Defeat
			Virtue	:	Vice
Violent	:	Gentle	**Visible**	:	Invisible
Visitor	:	Host	**Voluntary**	:	Compulsory
Voluntary	:	Involuntary			

W

War	:	Peace	**Winter**	:	Summer
Warm	:	Cool	**To work**	:	To rest
To waste	:	To save	**Woman**	:	man
Water	:	Land	**Women**	:	men
Weak	:	Powerful, strong	**Worse**	:	Better
			Worst	:	Best
Wealth	:	Poverty	**Wrong**	:	Correct, right
Wealthy	:	Poor	**Wax**	:	Wane
Wedding	:	Divorce	**Weak**	:	Strong
Well	:	Ill	**Wet**	:	Dry
Wet	:	Dry	**White**	:	Black
White	:	Black	**Wide**	:	Narrow
Whole	:	Part	**Win**	:	Lose
Wide	:	Narrow	**Wisdom**	:	Folly, stupidity
Wife	:	Husband	**Within**	:	Outside
To win	:	To lose			
Winner	:	Loser			

Y,Z

Yes	:	No		**Zip**	:	Unzip
Yin	:	Yang		**Zenith**	:	Nadir

MULTIPLE CHOICE QUESTIONS

SYNONYMS

Choose the correct Synonym or Meaning of the given Word from the options provided below in each case.

1. **Corpulent**
   a) Lean　　　　b) Gaunt
   c) Emaciated　d) Obese

2. **Embezzle**
   a) Misappropriate　b) Balance
   c) Remunerate　　　d) Clear

3. **Brief**
   a) Limited　b) Small
   c) Little　　d) Short

4. **Vent**
   a) Opening　b) Stodge
   c) End　　　d) Forgone

5. **August**
   a) Common　　b) Ridiculous
   c) Dignified　d) Petty

6. **Canny**
   a) Obstinate　b) Handsome
   c) Clever　　　d) Stout

7. **Alert**
   a) Energetic　　b) Observant
   c) Intelligent　d) Watchful

8. **Warrior**
   a) Soldier　b) Sailor
   c) Pirate　　d) Spy

9. **Adversity**
   a) Misfortune　b) Crisis
   c) Failure　　　d) Helplessness

10. **Distant**
   a) Reserved　b) Far
   c) Removed　　d) Separate

11. **Fake**
   a) Original　　　b) Imitation
   c) Trustworthy　d) Loyal

12. **Indict**
   a) Condemn　b) Reprimand
   c) Accuse　　d) Allege

13. **Stringent**
   a) Dry　　　　b) Strained
   c) Rigorous　d) Shrill

14. **Lament**
   a) Complain　b) Comment
   c) Condone　　d) Console

15. **Hesitated**
   a) Stopped　b) Paused
   c) Slowed　　d) Postponed

16. **Rescue**
   a) Command　b) Help
   c) Defence　　d) Safety

17. **Attempt**
   a) Try　　　b) Serve
   c) Explain　d) Explore

18. **Foray**
   a) Intuition　b) Ranger
   c) Contest　　d) Maraud

19. **Reckless**
   a) Courageous　b) Rash
   c) Bold　　　　d) Daring

20. **Inebriate**
   a) Dreamy　b) Stupefied
   c) Drunken　d) Unsteady

21. **Consequences**
   a) Conclusions　b) Results
   c) Difficulties　d) Applications

22. **Improvement**
   a) Preference　b) Promotion
   c) Advancement　d) Betterment

23. **Ironic**
   a) Inflexible　　b) Bitter
   c) Good-natured　d) Sarcastic

24. **Moving**
   a) Taking　b) Toying
   c) Shifting　d) Turning

25. Abject
a) Challenge   b) Miserable
c) Deny   d) Disobey

26. Sterile
a) Barren   b) Arid
c) Childless   d) Dry

27. Timid
a) Fast   b) Slow
c) Medium   d) Shy

28. Extricate
a) Pull   b) Free
c) Tie   d) Complicate

29. Neutral
a) Unbiased   b) Undecided
c) Non-aligned   d) Indifferent

30. Shallow
a) Artificial   b) Superficial
c) Foolish   d) Worthless

31. Diversion
a) Amusement   b) Distortion
c) Deviation   d) Bylane

32. Insolvent
a) Poor   b) Bankrupt
c) Penniless   d) Broke

33. Inexplicable
a) Confusing   b) Unaccountable
c) Chaotic   d) Unconnected

34. Feeble
a) Weak   b) Vain
c) Arrogant   d) Sick

35. Transient
a) Transparent   b) Fleeting
c) Feeble   d) Fanciful

36. Bare
a) Uncovered   b) Tolerate
c) Clear   d) Neat

37. Repeal
a) Sanction   b) Perpetuate
c) Pass   d) Cancel

38. Salacity
a) Bliss   b) Depression
c) Indecency   d) Recession

39. Ecstatic
a) Animated   b) Bewildered
c) Enraptured   d) Contested

40. Admonish
a) Punish   b) Curse
c) Dismiss   d) Reprimand

41. Diligent
a) Progressive   b) Brilliant
c) Inventive   d) Hard-working

42. Pious
a) Pure   b) Pretentious
c) Clean   d) Devout

43. Browse
a) Heal   b) Deceive
c) Examine   d) Strike

44. Infrequent
a) Never   b) Usual
c) Rare   d) Sometimes

45. Restraint
a) Hindrance   b) Repression
c) Obstacle   d) Restriction

46. Deify
a) Flatter   b) Worship
c) Challenge   d) Face

47. Harbinger
a) Messenger   b) Steward
c) Forerunner   d) Pilot

48. Venue
a) Place   b) Agenda
c) Time   d) Duration

49. Candid
a) Apparent   b) Explicit
c) Frank   d) Bright

50. Meld
a) Soothe   b) Merge
c) Purchase   d) Glisten

51. Lynch
  a) Hang
  b) Madden
  c) Kill
  d) Shoot

52. Torture
  a) Torment
  b) Chastisement
  c) Harassment
  d) Terror

53. Abundant
  a) Ripe
  b) Cheap
  c) Plenty
  d) Absent

54. Entire
  a) Part
  b) Quarter
  c) Whole
  d) Half

55. Destitution
  a) Humility
  b) Moderation
  c) Poverty
  d) Begging

56. Wretched
  a) Poor
  b) Foolish
  c) Insane
  d) Strained

57. Intimidate
  a) Hint
  b) Frighten
  c) Bluff
  d) Harass

58. Cantankerous
  a) Quarrelsome
  b) Rash
  c) Disrespectful
  d) Noisy

59. Rant
  a) Praise
  b) Formalize
  c) Complain
  d) Scorn

60. Zany
  a) Clown
  b) Pet
  c) Thief
  d) magician

61. Taciturnity
  a) Dumbness
  b) Changeableness
  c) Hesitation
  d) Reserve

62. Massacre
  a) Murder
  b) Stab
  c) Assassinate
  d) Slaughter

63. Ken
  a) Ignorance
  b) Witness
  c) trial
  d) Knowledge

64. Wary
  a) sad
  b) Vigilant
  c) Distorted
  d) Tired

65. Rabble
  a) Mob
  b) Noise
  c) Roar
  d) Rubbish

66. Mayhem
  a) Jubilation
  b) havoc
  c) Excitement
  d) Defeat

67. Ponder
  a) Think
  b) Evaluate
  c) Anticipate
  d) Increase

68. Connoisseur
  a) Ignorant
  b) Lover of art
  c) Interpreter
  d) Delinquent

69. Shiver
  a) Feel
  b) Rock
  c) Tremble
  d) Move

70. Prestige
  a) Influence
  b) Quality
  c) name
  d) Wealth

71. Stringent
  a) Tense
  b) Stringly
  c) Strict
  d) Shrink

72. Insomnia
  a) Lethargy
  b) Sleeplessness
  c) Drunkenness
  d) Unconsciousness

73. Laud
  a) Lord
  b) Eulogy
  c) Praise
  d) Extolled

74. Repercussion
  a) Clever reply
  b) recollection
  c) Remuneration
  d) Reaction

75. Impromptu
  a) Offhand
  b) Unimportant
  c) Unreal
  d) Effective

76. Frugality
  a) Foolishness
  b) Extremity
  c) Enthusiasm
  d) Economy

77. Correspondence
a) Agreements   b) Contracts
c) Documents   d) Letters

78. Ascend
a) Leap   b) Grow
c) Deviate   d) Mount

79. Furore
a) Excitement   b) Worry
c) Flux   d) Change

80. Synopsis
a) Index   b) Mixture
c) Summary   d) Puzzles

81. Turn up
a) Land up   b) Show up
c) Crop up   d) Come up

82. Vigour
a) Strength   b) Boldness
c) Warmth   d) Enthusiasm

83. Garnish
a) Paint   b) Garner
c) Adorn   d) Abuse

84. Mendacious
a) Confident   b) False
c) Encouraging   d) Provocative

85. Garrulity
a) Credulity   b) Senility
c) Loquaciousness   d) Speciousness

86. Morose
a) Annoyed   b) Gloomy
c) Moody   d) Displeased

87. Voraciousness
a) truthful   b) Gluttonous
c) Funny   d) Venturous

88. Awakened
a) Enlightened   b) Realized
c) Shook   d) Waken

89. Gratify
a) Appreciate   b) Frank
c) Indulge   d) Pacify

90. Precarious
a) Cautious   b) critical
c) Perilous   d) Brittle

91. Infamy
a) Dishonour   b) Glory
c) Integrity   d) Reputation

92. Masterly
a) Crafty   b) Skilful
c) Meaningful   d) Cruel

93. Scintillating
a) Smouldering   b) Glittering
c) Touching   d) Warming

94. Tepid
a) Hot   b) Warm
c) Cold   d) Boiling

95. Voracious
a) Wild   b) Greedy
c) Angry   d) Quick

96. Unite
a) Unfold   b) Unchain
c) Combine   d) Unhinge

97. Combat
a) Conflict   b) Quarrel
c) Feud   d) Fight

98. Refectory
a) Restaurant   b) Parlour
c) Living room   d) Dining room

99. Uncouth
a) Ungraceful   b) Rough
c) Slovenly   d) Dirty

100. Error
a) Misadventure   b) Misgiving
c) Ambiguity   d) Blunder

101. Commensurate
a) Measurable   b) Proportionate
c) Beginning   d) Appropriate

102. Debacle
a) Collapse   b) Decline
c) Defeat   d) Disgrace

103. Germane
a) Responsible
b) Logical
c) Possible
d) Relevant

104. Distinction
a) Diffusion
b) Disagreement
c) Different
d) Degree

105. Retain
a) Keep
b) Recall
c) Preserve
d) Conserve

106. Vicissitudes
a) Sorrows
b) Misfortunes
c) Changes
d) Surprises

107. Insatiable
a) Unsatisfiable
b) Unchanging
c) Irreconcilable
d) Undesirable

108. Nimble
a) Unrhythmic
b) Lively
c) Quickening
d) Clear

109. Bohemian
a) Hostile
b) Unconventional
c) Sinister
d) Unfriendly

110. Fatal
a) Grievous
b) Dangerous
c) Serious
d) Deadly

111. Callous
a) Passive
b) Unkind
c) Cursed
d) Unfeeling

112. Headway
a) Progress
b) Thinking
c) Efforts
d) Start

113. Fabricated
a) Forged
b) Historical
c) Prepared
d) Genuine

114. Manifest
a) Easily perceived
b) Easily acquired
c) Easily infected
d) Easily deflected

115. Lapse
a) Trick
b) Interval
c) Error
d) Ignorance

116. Dismal
a) Poor
b) Sorrowful
c) Minimum
d) Short

117. Subsequent
a) Later
b) Many
c) Few
d) Earlier

118. Pioneers
a) Inventors
b) Explorers
c) Colonialist
d) Settlers

119. Propensity
a) Natural tendency
b) Aptitude
c) Characteristic
d) Quality

120. Sanguine
a) Depressed
b) Pessimistic
c) Anxious
d) Optimistic

121. Averse
a) Convinced
b) Angry
c) Agreeable
d) Opposed

122. Outwitted
a) Defeated
b) Befooled
c) Cheated
d) Outmanoeuvred

123. Mandatory
a) Compulsory
b) Necessary
c) Required
d) Needed

124. Amity
a) Bondage
b) Contention
c) Friendship
d) Understanding

125. Exceptional
a) Avoidable
b) Unusual
c) Strange
d) Abnormal

126. Mud-slinging
a) Caricatures
b) Mockery
c) Slander
d) Quarelling

127. Precisely
a) Approximately
b) Exactly
c) Accurately
d) Concisely

128. **Preposterous**
   a) Heartless   b) Impractical
   c) Absurd   d) Abnormal

129. **Languishing**
   a) Convicted   b) Suffering
   c) Attempting   d) Avoiding

130. **Inebriated**
   a) Inexperienced   b) Tired
   c) Befuddled   d) Intoxicated

131. **Incoherent**
   a) Irrational   b) Inconsistent
   c) Irrelevant   d) Irritating

132. **Abstruse**
   a) Dangerous   b) Impractical
   c) Obscure   d) Irrational

133. **Internecine**
   a) Mutually
   b) Baneful, destructive
   c) Pernicious
   d) Detrimental

134. **Obstreperous**
   a) Sullen   b) Unruly
   c) Lazy   d) Awkward

135. **Credible**
   a) Believable   b) False
   c) Readable   d) Praiseworthy

136. **Environment**
   a) nationality   b) Heredity
   c) Nature   d) Surroundings

137. **Garrulous**
   a) Talks a lot   b) Laughs a lot
   c) Giggles   d) Repeats gossip
      all the time

138. **Aberration**
   a) Procrastination   b) Privilege
   c) Deviation   d) Steadfastness

139. **Lamentable**
   a) Unpardonable   b) Deplorable
   c) Inexcusable   d) Terrible

140. **Rupture**
   a) Break   b) Damage
   c) Breach   d) Gap

141. **Sea-change**
   a) Complete change
   b) Partial change
   c) Favourable change
   d) Unfavourable change

142. **Gullible**
   a) Fallible   b) Enthusiastic
   c) Unsuspecting   d) Unrealistic

143. **Sane**
   a) Rational   b) Obscure
   c) Wild   d) Arrogant

144. **Vandalism**
   a) Disturbance   b) Ravage
   c) Provocation   d) Violence

145. **Come a round**
   a) Recover   b) Walk
   c) Move   d) Eat

146. **Alien**
   a) Foreign   b) Extraneous
   c) Unusual   d) Exotic

147. **Hazardous**
   a) Tricky   b) Harmful
   c) Difficult   d) Dangerous

148. **Vigilant**
   a) Intelligent   b) Ambitious
   c) Watchful   d) Smart

149. **Lately**
   a) Immediately   b) Early
   c) Recently   d) Late

150. **Extinct**
   a) Aggresive   b) Non-existent
   c) Scattered   d) Feeble

151. **Alleviated**
   a) Mitigated   b) Moderated
   c) Removed   d) Lightened

152. Credentials
a) Principles
b) Dependability
c) Capacity to return loans
d) Trustworthiness

153. Impending
a) Threatening
b) Imminent
c) Terrible
d) Possible

154. Relieve
a) Alleviate
b) Mitigate
c) Moderate
d) Abate

155. Illicit
a) Indigenous
b) Illegitimate
c) Illegal
d) Country

156. Proselytise
a) Translate
b) Hypnotise
c) Attack
d) Convert

157. Graphic
a) Picture
b) Drawing
c) Vivid
d) Broad

158. Testimonials
a) Witnesses
b) Testaments
c) Tokens
d) Credentials

159. Attribute
a) Infer
b) Impute
c) Inhere
d) Inundate

160. Lynched
a) Beaten up
b) Captured
c) Killed
d) Mutilated

161. Compromise
a) Adjust
b) Accommodate
c) Yield
d) Conciliate

162. Indifference
a) Disinterest
b) Concern
c) Displeasure
d) Caution

163. Mettle
a) Persistence
b) Strength
c) Courage
d) Heroism

164. Eulogised
a) Appreciated
b) Praised
c) Approved
d) Applauded

165. Rewarding
a) Profitable
b) Paying
c) Serviceable
d) Precious

166. Benevolence
a) Ill-will
b) Kindness
c) Morbidity
d) Vision

167. Verdict
a) Judgement
b) Voice
c) Outcome
d) Prediction

168. Lucrative
a) Tempting
b) Attractive
c) Profitable
d) Honourable

169. Incensed
a) Excited
b) Inflamed
c) Enraged
d) Enthused

170. Lucid
a) Elaborate
b) Clear
c) Noble
d) Intricate

171. Sycophants
a) Submissive
b) Foppish
c) Flatterers
d) Eager

172. Outset
a) End
b) Beginning
c) Middle
d) Entrance

173. Emulate
a) Imitate
b) Modify
c) Mollify
d) Inhabit

174. Oblivious
a) Precarious
b) Unmindful
c) Aware
d) Watchful

175. Fictitious
a) Unbelievable
b) Unreliable
c) Infamous
d) Unreal

176. Anxiety
a) Curiosity
b) Grief
c) Uneasiness
d) Eagerness

177. Corroborated
a) Confirmed   b) Disproved
c) Condemned   d) Seconded

178. Comely
a) Delightful   b) Pretty
c) Homely   d) Elegant

179. Capricious
a) Misleading   b) Whimsical
c) Erratic   d) Unpredictable

180. Neglected
a) Refused   b) Failed
c) Promised   d) Obstructed

181. Enmeshed
a) Entangled   b) Hit
c) Struck   d) Ensured

182. Baffled
a) Defeated   b) Thwarted
c) Foiled   d) Circumvented

183. Scandal
a) Silly notion   b) Talk
c) Rumour   d) Disgraceful
                        action

184. Industrious
a) Energetic   b) Prompt
c) Excellent   d) Diligent

185. Headstrong
a) Thick-headed   b) Obstinate
c) Robust   d) Witty

186. Spontaneous
a) Well-timed   b) Willing
c) Instinctive   d) Instantaneous

187. Deprecated
a) Welcomed   b) Denied
c) Protested   d) Humiliated

188. Lucrative
a) Good   b) Profitable
c) Excellent   d) Significant

189. Licentious
a) Libertine   b) Loafer
c) Criminal   d) Freelance

190. Approbation
a) Understanding   b) Approval
c) Admiration   d) Appreciation

191. Sprightly
a) Beautiful   b) Lively
c) Intelligent   d) Sporty

192. Rights
a) Status   b) Truth
c) Virtues   d) Privileges

193. Stood up to
a) Challenged   b) Fought back
c) Resisted   d) Defeated

194. Transparent
a) Verbose   b) Involved
c) Lucid   d) Witty

195. Annihilated
a) Dismembered   b) Reduced
c) Destroyed   d) Split

196. Exemplary
a) Suitable   b) Clear
c) Elementary   d) Admirable

197. Misogynism
a) Hate for men   b) Hate for women
c) Love for men   d) Love for women

198. Indiscriminate
a) Desperate   b) Undifferentiated
c) Discreet   d) Insensitive

199. Lethargy
a) Serenity   b) Impassivity
c) Laxity   d) Listlessness

200. Prognosis
a) Scheme   b) Forcast
c) Preface   d) Identification

201. Emaciated
a) Very thin   b) Very aged
c) Very tall   d) Very sleepy

202. Contract
a) Tract   b) Give
c) Expand   d) Abridge

203. Inedible
   a) Unfit for human consumption
   b) Pollutent
   c) Vitiated
   d) Eatable

204. Docile
   a) Vague   b) Gentle
   c) Stupid   d) Stubborn

205. Enigmatic
   a) Displeased   b) Puzzling
   c) Learned   d) Short-sighted

206. Homage
   a) Excessive
   b) Show respect, humility and
      reverance
   c) Poverty
   d) Flattery

207. Virile
   a) Athletic   b) Pompous
   c) Manly   d) Bashful

208. Fiasco
   a) Failure   b) Festival
   c) Disaster   d) Misfortune

209. Nostalgic
   a) Indolent   b) Diseased
   c) Homesick   d) Soothing

210. Sporadic
   a) Epidemic   b) Whirling
   c) Occasional   d) Stagnant

211. Ostentatious
   a) Wealthy   b) Talkative
   c) Showy   d) Noisy

212. Histrionic
   a) Hypersensitive
   b) Overdramatic
   c) Historically
   d) Inactive

213. Arbiter
   a) Very bitter
   b) A priest
   c) A despot
   d) One appointed by two parties to
      settle a dispute

214. Didactic
   a) Blunt
   b) In poetic metre
   c) Direct
   d) Of the nature of teaching

215. Baton
   a) Cargo
   b) Cane
   c) Stick used in conducting an orchestra
   d) Drumstick

216. Buoyancy
   a) Child-like   b) Sturdy
   c) Brisk   d) Light-hearted

217. Unalloyed
   a) Not connected   b) Calm
   c) Pure   d) Inferior

218. Debonair
   a) Superficial   b) Very stylish
   c) Pleasant   d) Flighty

219. Solecism
   a) Wise saying
   b) Witty quip
   c) Clever argument
   d) Grammatical error

220. Corroborate
   a) Collaborate   b) Substantiate
   c) Narrate   d) Correlate

221. Delirious
   a) Delicious   b) Pleasing
   c) Desperate   d) Excited

222. Licentious
   a) Immoral   b) Intellectual
   c) Moral   d) Without license

223. **Squander**
   a) Expansive　　b) waste
   c) Litter　　d) Economical

224. **Circuitous**
   a) Indirect　　b) Confusing
   c) Crooked　　d) Cyclic

225. **Immune**
   a) Hostile　　b) Disturbing
   c) Statutory　　d) Exempt

226. **Ideal**
   a) Thorough　　b) Civilised
   c) Useless　　d) Perfect

227. **Acronym**
   a) Similar meaning
   b) Poem of sorrow
   c) Word formed from abbreviation
   d) Pen name used by author

228. **Acumen**
   a) Knowledge　　b) Bitterness
   c) Abundance　　d) Deficit

229. **Extinct**
   a) No longer in existence
   b) Dull
   c) Wonderful
   d) Still in existence

230. **Incompatible**
   a) Reasonable　　b) Capable
   c) Contradictory　　d) Faulty

231. **Reiterate**
   a) Illustrate　　b) Repeat
   c) Deny　　d) Receipt

232. **Give in**
   a) Give　　b) Receive
   c) Distribute　　d) Yield

233. **Give up**
   a) Give　　b) Stop doing
   c) Start　　d) Start doing

234. **Fictitious**
   a) False　　b) Foul
   c) Fraud　　d) Flattering

235. **Cache**
   a) Hiding place　　b) Tide
   c) Lock　　d) Automobile

236. **Handful**
   a) Few or little　　b) Powerless
   c) Useless　　d) Powerful

237. **Rigid**
   a) Sticky　　b) Hard
   c) Solid　　d) Bent

238. **Rejoice**
   a) Rebuild　　b) Rename
   c) Delight　　d) Lighten

239. **Cryptic**
   a) Silence　　b) A puzzle
   c) Precise　　d) Vault

240. **Effusion**
   a) Exclamation　　b) Shocking
   c) Pouring forth　　d) Threatening

241. **Emanciated**
   a) Exist　　b) Restrain
   c) Set free　　d) Correct morally

242. **Enigma**
   a) Reply　　b) Puzzling
   c) Praise　　d) Sharp

243. **Contingency**
   a) Conditionality　　b) Originality
   c) Independence　　d) Autonomous

244. **Gluttony**
   a) Sadness　　b) Greedy
   c) Beatitude　　d) Satisfaction

245. **Eulogistic**
   a) Practical　　b) Wanderer
   c) Prank　　d) Praising

246. **Abortive**
   a) Unsuccessful　　b) Failure
   c) Consuming　　d) Fruitful

247. **Emulate**
   a) Deny　　b) Question
   c) Imitate　　d) Discuss

248. Coup
a) Small enclosure b) Accident
c) Sudden overthrow d) Clever reply
of a government

249. Parasite
a) Disease b) One that clings
c) Loss of motion d) Exterminator

250. Cite
a) Point out b) Quote
c) see clearly d) memorise

251. Starve
a) Naked b) Crawl
c) Hungry d) Naughty

252. Dexterity
a) Zest b) Skill
c) Tempo d) Efficiency

253. Bountiful
a) Generous b) Shameful
c) Pretty d) Rude

254. Nascent
a) Crude b) Initial
c) Unpleasant d) Latest

255. Interim
a) Timely b) Interval
c) Temporary d) Internal

256. Hypothetical
a) Based on supposition
b) Double faced
c) Methodical
d) Practical

257. Obliterate
a) Blot out b) Block up
c) Slow down d) Decline

258. Reminiscent
a) Remembrance b) Revival
c) Remembered d) Reminding one

259. Notoriety
a) Unpleasant experience
b) Unfavourably known
c) Public shame
d) Wrong option

260. Mottle
a) mark with spot b) Spoil
c) Erase d) Colour

261. Privy
a) Quiet b) Secretive
c) Dishonest d) Cautious

262. Hallowed
a) Mellowed b) Old
c) Decayed d) Sacred

263. Glean
a) Speak b) Polish
c) Gather bit by bit d) Discover

264. Festal
a) Noisy b) Sad
c) Serious d) Merry

265. Vituperate
a) Abuse b) Encourage
c) Appraise d) Appreciate

266. Alacrity
a) Suspicion b) Unwillingly
c) Hesitatingly d) Eagerness

267. Sonorous
a) Loud b) Sleepy
c) Heavy d) Bright

268. Genesis
a) Beginning b) Movement
c) Relevant d) Style

269. Trumpery
a) Trick b) Treasure
c) Rubbish
d) Useless argument

270. Incredulous
a) Skeptical b) Superstitious
c) Unreliable d) Unimaginable

271. Catharsis
a) Anti-climax
b) Sudden happening
c) Outlet for strong emotion
d) Informal discussion

272. Obscure
a) Unknown   b) Famous
c) Well known   d) Prevalent

273. Cacophony
a) Dance   b) Rooster
c) Applause   d) Discordant

274. Breach
a) Restrict   b) Break
c) Slander   d) Rift

275. Remorse
a) Reliant   b) Regret
c) Vehement   d) Voluble

276. Gall
a) Poison   b) Taste
c) Nerve   d) Bitterness

277. Braggadocio
a) Empty boasting b) Misadventure
c) Sad plight   d) Bribery

278. Bovine
a) Dimwitted   b) Meat extract
c) Like an ox   d) An expert

279. Lachrymose
a) Impious   b) Mournful
c) Unimpressive d) Moist

280. Gargoyle
a) Creature   b) Garish
c) Golden eagle d) Stone spout

281. Bigamy
a) Having more   b) Biblical
than one wife   reference
or husband
c) Ambiguity   d) Concern

282. Myriad
a) Imaginary   b) Bright
c) A great number d) variety

283. Cavil
a) Quibble   b) Amuse
c) Appreciate   d) Munch

284. Cynosure
a) Threat
b) Rejoice
c) Centre of attraction
d) Rebel

285. Pastel
a) dark shade   b) Conflict
c) Attempt   d) Light shade

286. Façade
a) Aspect
b) Hilly view
c) Exact copy
d) Front of a building

287. Wreak
a) Inflict   b) Sweat
c) Unpleasant   d) Twist

288. Accolade
a) Drink   b) Balcony
c) Honour   d) Fruit

289. Hearty
a) Cold   b) Warm
c) Warmly   d) Cordially

290. Glitter
a) Shining   b) Bright
c) Gleams   d) Gleaming

291. Several
a) A few   b) Some
c) Many   d) A lot of

292. Quarrel
a) Chat   b) Dispute
c) Disputes   d) Altercation

293. Partial
a) Fairless   b) Unequal
c) Favouring   d) Biased

294. Spacious
a) Small   b) Large
c) Cramped   d) Limited

295. Indecent
a) Bad   b) Ugly
c) Vulgar   d) Indelicately

296. Fiction
   a) Essay   b) Fact
   c) Story   d) Reality

297. Probable
   a) Like   b) Likely
   c) Presume   d) Clear

298. Kind
   a) Warm   b) Cruel
   c) Style   d) Sad

299. Trickling
   a) Dripping   b) Crawling
   c) Gushing   d) Pouring

300. Immediately
   a) Hastily   b) At once
   c) Belatedly   d) Slowly

301. Cultivate
   a) Develop   b) Change
   c) Trained   d) Teach

302. Exhausted
   a) Dull   b) Brisk
   c) Ill   d) Tired

303. Weather
   a) Report   b) Climate
   c) Reason   d) Sky

304. Fragile
   a) Weak   b) Weaker
   c) Strong   d) Soundless

305. Remote
   a) Far   b) Rare
   c) Nearly   d) Distant

306. Humility
   a) Bashful   b) Shyness
   c) Modesty   d) Humbleness

307. Ceased
   a) Seized   b) Stopped
   c) Reduce   d) Seizure

308. Probable
   a) Likely   b) Like
   c) Presume   d) Clear

309. Strict
   a) Severe   b) Tough
   c) Softly   d) Lenient

310. Loyal
   a) Disloyal   b) Truly
   c) Faithful   d) Loyalty

311. Lovely
   a) Fairly   b) Charming
   c) Charmless   d) Lovingly

312. Royal
   a) Regal   b) Great
   c) Noble   d) Prince

313. Liberal
   a) Greedy   b) Free
   c) Generous   d) Generosity

314. Absent
   a) Missing   b) Variety
   c) Clamour   d) Glamour

315. Accurate
   a) Enclosure   b) Zenith
   c) Totality   d) Correct

316. Admit
   a) Allow   b) Come
   c) Gone   d) Rosy

317. Alive
   a) Living   b) Scatter
   c) Caramel   d) Tresspass

318. Ally
   a) Friend   b) Enemy
   c) Capital   d) Bubble

319. Ancient
   a) Crease   b) Past
   c) Modern   d) Old

320. Apart
   a) Separate   b) Sanguine
   c) Banal   d) Crazy

321. Ablaze
   a) Unexcited   b) Dark
   c) Dim   d) Ignited

322. Accost
a) Scorn b) Shun
c) Confront d) Dodge

323. Adapt
a) Modify b) Dejected
c) Adjourn d) Defer

324. Adept
a) Aching b) Conform
c) Adapt d) Skilled

325. Astute
a) Culmination b) Abduct
c) Grab d) Intelligent

326. Abject
a) Wretched b) Capable
c) Expert d) Astute

327. Adjourn
a) Seize b) Delay
c) Accord d) Deal

328. Accord
a) Deplorable b) Base
c) Concord d) Brace

329. Accost
a) Alter b) Order
c) Confront d) Adjoin

330. Adjudge
a) Pact b) Harmony
c) Decide d) Join

331. Acquit
a) Impress b) Apex
c) Climax d) Liberate

332. Adjust
a) Transform b) Sore
c) Throbbing d) Accommodate

333. Adjoin
a) Connect b) Max
c) Snatch d) Crafty

334. Avouch
a) Abject b) Discontinue
c) Harmony d) Affirm

335. Aplomb
a) Adjudge b) Adjudicate
c) Consider d) Poise

336. Accept
a) Nagging b) Adept
c) Accomplished d) Welcome

337. Affirm
a) Confirm b) Accost
c) Annoy d) Entice

338. Abduct
a) Kidnap b) Non-chalance
c) Tact d) Balance

339. Acumen
a) Wisdom b) Determine
c) Acquit d) Vindicate

340. Aching
a) Hurting b) Brilliance
c) Alter d) Convert

341. Amaze
a) Bewilder b) Avouch
c) Admit d) Avow

342. Apex
a) Pinnacle b) Perplex
c) Acumen d) Intellect

343. Stringent
a) Stern b) Civilized
c) Hail d) Blast

344. Accurate
a) Dribble b) Arid
c) Desert d) Reliable

345. Frugality
a) Thrift b) Approval
c) Dispel d) Exile

346. Vindicate
a) Explain b) Evil
c) Sinister d) Repay

347. Distaste
a) Hatred b) Annex
c) Anchored d) Approval

348. Voracious
a) Censure   b) Rise
c) Lift   d) Ravenous

349. Admiration
a) Esteem   b) Badge
c) Decline   d) Stun

350. Admiration
a) Esteem   b) Badge
c) Decline   d) Stun

351. Curtail
a) Address   b) Bewilder
c) Auspicious   d) Downsize

352. Afloat
a) Drifting   b) Accept
c) Refusal   d) Stoppage

353. Home
a) Requite   b) Forgive
c) Antipathy   d) Domicile

354. Distinction
a) Honor   b) Credible
c) Convincing   d) Corrupt

355. Climb
a) Punish   b) Allergy
c) Respect   d) Mounting

356. Mystify
a) Puzzle   b) Dispassionate
c) Awe   d) Wonder

357. Harmful
a) Disregard   b) Lessen
c) Abbreviate   d) Deadly

358. Flinch
a) Recoil   b) Unmoored
c) Loose   d) Sanctuary

359. Boycott
a) Eager   b) Ardent
c) Expand   d) Prohibition

360. Dismiss
a) Deport   b) Allow
c) Rough   d) Boorish

361. Cruel
a) Resist   b) Refuse
c) Fruitful   d) Inhuman

362. Shower
a) Storm   b) Avidity
c) Greediness   d) Generosity

363. Desolate
a) Harsh   b) Rigid
c) Extravagant d) Empty

364. Aid
a) Help   b) Original
c) Fervent   d) Exhausting

365. Bottomless
a) Dignified   b) Scam
c) Abstinent   d) Endless

366. Astonish
a) Shock   b) Desire
c) Pay   d) Announce

367. Disturb
a) Heighten   b) Prophet
c) Stern   d) Alter

368. Belittle
a) Debase   b) Reliable
c) Avidity   d) Repay

369. Despise
a) Facet   b) Gutty
c) Loud   d) Detest

370. Cutting
a) caustic   b) Antipathy
c) Eager   d) Awe

371. Quit
a) Lessen   b) Unmoored
c) Sanctuary   d) Cease

372. Complex
a) Complicated b) Approval
c) Rise   d) Puzzle

373. Ample
a) Deadly   b) Resist
c) Refusal   d) Sufficient

374. Highlight
a) Emphasize   b) Dispel
c) Inhuman   d) Shower

375. Aide
a) Clothes   b) Deadly
c) Resist   d) Associate

376. Angry
a) Cutting   b) Facet
c) Gutty   d) Loud

377. Keen
a) Shower   b) Arid
c) Citadel   d) Astute

378. Determined
a) Insistent   b) Resist
c) Refusal   d) Dispel

379. Comply
a) Lessen   b) Unmoored
c) Sanctuary   d) Heed

380. Advise
a) Berate   b) Dispel
c) Inhuman   d) Shower

381. Beautify
a) Shower   b) Arid
c) Citadel   d) Grace

382. Adept
a) Clever   b) Facet
c) Gutty   d) Loud

383. Applause
a) Antipathy   b) Eager
c) Awe   d) Flattery

384. Calamity
a) Mishap   b) Scam
c) Abstinent   d) Endless

385. Backing
a) Help   b) Original
c) Fervent   d) Assistance

386. Pleasant
a) Amiable   b) Aid
c) Exhausting   d) Bottomless

387. Artistic
a) Announce   b) Disturb
c) Heighten   d) Creative

388. Affection
a) Sympathy   b) Prophet
c) Stern   d) Alter

389. Disease
a) Bottomless   b) Dignified
c) Astonish   d) Calamity

390. Moneyed
a) Upscale   b) Belittle
c) Debase   d) Reliable

391. Rapid
a) Prophet   b) Stern
c) Alter   d) Quick

392. Alertness
a) Eagerness   b) Reliable
c) Avidity   d) Repay

393. Disaffect
a) Gutty   b) Loud
c) Detest   d) Separate

394. Charge
a) Recount   b) Reliable
c) Avidity   d) Repay

395. Adherence
a) Despise   b) Facet
c) Gutty   d) Faithfulness

396. Ease
a) Allay   b) Complicated
c) Approval   d) Rise

397. Advert
a) Unmoored   b) Sanctuary
c) Cease   d) Insinuate

398. Detached
a) Distant   b) Highlight
c) Emphasize   d) Dispel

399. Charitable
a) Clothes   b) Deadly
c) Resist   d) Humanitarian

400. Enigmatic
a) Opaque   b) Angry
c) Cutting   d) Facet

401. Contradictory
a) Uncertain b) Dispel
c) Charitable d) Clothes

402. Affable
a) Reliable   b) Avidity
c) Repay   d) Lovable

403. Amiable
a) Polite   b) Humanitarian
c) Enigmatic d) Opaque

404. Abundant
a) Awe   b) Quit
c) Lessen   d) Spacious

405. Acrimony
a) Bitterness b) Gutty
c) Loud   d) Detest

406. Crush
a) Angry   b) Cutting
c) Facet   d) Decimate

407. Aberration
a) Deviation b) Emphasize
c) Dispel   d) Charitable

408. Unidentified
a) Resist   b) Humanitarian
c) Enigmatic d) Unacknowledged

409. Assume
a) Await   b) Advert
c) Unmoored   d) Sanctuary

410. Animosity
a) Detached   b) Distant
c) Highlight d) Distaste

411. Lethargy
a) Unconcern b) Opaque
c) Angry   d) Cutting

412. Disposition
a) caustic   b) Antipathy
c) Eager   d) Leaning

413. Irresponsible
a) Capricious b) Repay
c) Despise   d) Facet

414. Esoteric
a) Antipathy b) Eager
c) Awe   d) Mystic

415. Ancient
a) Old-fashioned b) Approval
c) Rise   d) Puzzle

416. Form
a) Reliable   b) Avidity
c) Repay   d) Original

417. Avid
a) Fervent   b) Charge
c) Recount   d) Reliable

418. Uphill
a) Ease   b) Allay
c) Complicated d) Exhausting

419. Noble
a) Dignified b) Loud
c) Detest   d) Separate

420. Gimmick
a) Adherence b) Despise
c) Facet   d) Scam

421. Adversity
a) Scourge   b) Abstinent
c) Endless   d) Backing

422. Inexperienced
a) Announce   b) Disturb
c) Heighten   d) Jellybean

423. Blunt
a) Forthright b) Exhausting
c) Bottomless d) Artistic

424. Relent
a) Creative   b) Affection
c) Sympathy   d) Bow

425. Arbitrary
a) Unstable   b) Original
c) Fervent   d) Assistance

426. Berate
a) Heighten   b) Prophet
c) Stern   d) Rebuke

427. Abrasive
a) Acerbic   b) Disease
c) Bottomless   d) Dignified

428. Discontinue
a) Repay   b) Disaffect
c) Gutty   d) Halt

429. Capitulate
a) Drop   b) Upscale
c) Belittle   d) Debase

430. Blow
a) Quick   b) Alertness
c) Eagerness   d) Crushing

431. Glamour
a) Dazzle   b) Insinuate
c) Detached   d) Distant

432. Flog
a) Adherence   b) Despise
c) Facet   d) Lash

433. Constant
a) Incurable   b) Advert
c) Unmoored   d) Sanctuary

434. Prudent
a) Distant   b) Highlight
c) Emphasize   d) Vigilant

435. Covert
a) Foxy   b) Complicated
c) Approval   d) Rise

436. Compassion
a) Stern   b) Alter
c) Quick   d) Forbearance

437. Clan
a) Mafia   b) Repay
c) Adherence   d) Despise

438. Duress
a) Reliable   b) Avidity
c) Repay   d) Constraint

439. Convincing
a) Compelling   b) Antipathy
c) Eager   d) Awe

440. Aprehensive
a) Quit   b) Lessen
c) Unmoored   d) Conscious

441. Avow
a) Maintain   b) Ample
c) Deadly   d) Resist

442. Balance
a) Approval   b) Rise
c) Puzzle   d) Poise

443. Welcome
a) Acquire   b) Resist
c) Refusal   d) Sufficient

444. Insist
a) Dispel   b) Charitable
c) Clothes   d) Assert

445. Seize
a) Snatch   b) Aid
c) Exhausting   d) Bottomless

446. Insight
a) Dignified   b) Astonish
c) Shock   d) Brilliance

447. Throbbing
a) Nagging   b) Heighten
c) Prophet   d) Stern

448. Daze
a) Announce   b) Disturb
c) Heighten   d) Impress

449. Max
a) Culmination   b) Help
c) Original   d) Fervent

450. Help
a) Abstinent   b) Endless
c) Backing   d) Guidance

451. Complete
a) Boundless   b) Creative
c) Affection   d) Sympathy

452. **Stagger**
   a) Dignified b) Astonish
   c) Calamity d) Confuse

453. **Change**
   a) Interest b) Prophet
   c) Stern d) Alter

454. **Diminish**
   a) Arid b) Citadel
   c) Grace d) Degrade

455. **Loathe**
   a) Scorn b) Determined
   c) Insistent d) Resist

456. **Annoying**
   a) Comply b) Lessen
   c) Unmoored d) Nasty

457. **Pass**
   a) Cease b) Resist
   c) Refusal d) Dispel

458. **Deep**
   a) Unmoored b) Sanctuary
   c) Heed d) Ideal

459. **Rich**
   a) Sufficient b) Arid
   c) Citadel d) Astute

460. **Underline**
   a) Deadly b) Resist
   c) Associate d) Underscore

461. **Belligerent**
   a) Aggressive b) Arid
   c) Citadel d) Grace

462. **Bemoan**
   a) Keen b) Shower
   c) Arid d) Deplore

463. **Bemused**
   a) Distracted b) Comply
   c) Lessen d) Unmoored

464. **Benign**
   a) Unmoored b) Sanctuary
   c) Heed d) Benevolent

465. **Benevolent**
   a) Caring b) Aide
   c) Clothes d) Deadly

466. **Berate**
   a) Insistent b) Resist
   c) Refusal d) Reproach

467. **Beseech**
   a) Implore b) Stern
   c) Alter d) Calamity

468. **Bestow**
   a) Help b) Original
   c) Fervent d) Lavish

469. **Bias**
   a) Penchant b) Affection
   c) Sympathy d) Prophet

470. **Bicker**
   a) Disease b) Bottomless
   c) Dignified d) Disagree

471. **Bifurcate**
   a) Divide b) Dignified
   c) Astonish d) Calamity

472. **Bilateral**
   a) Mishap b) Scam
   c) Abstinent d) Mutual

473. **Billowing**
   a) Undulate b) Assistance
   c) Pleasant d) Amiable

474. **Binge**
   a) Exhausting b) Bottomless
   c) Artistic d) Orgy

475. **Bland**
   a) Banal b) Alertness
   c) Eagerness d) Reliable

476. **Blare**
   a) Despise b) Facet
   c) Gutty d) Bark

477. **Blasphemy**
   a) Heresy b) Repay
   c) Adherence d) Despise

478. Bleak
a) Belittle   b) Debase
c) Reliable   d) Cold

479. Blatant
a) Outright   b) Faithfulness
c) Ease   d) Allay

480. Cogent
a) Eager   b) Awe
c) Flattery   d) Compelling

481. Confine
a) Imprison   b) Loud
c) Applause   d) Antipathy

482. Concurrent
a) Clever   b) Facet
c) Gutty   d) Simultaneous

483. Condone
a) Forgive   b) Citadel
c) Grace   d) Adept

484. Concord
a) Beautify   b) Shower
c) Arid   d) Harmony

485. Conclave
a) Gathering   b) Dispel
c) Inhuman   d) Shower

486. Concise
a) Heed   b) Advise
c) Berate   d) Brief

487. Concentric
a) Centred   b) Lessen
c) Unmoored   d) Sanctuary

488. Conceited
a) Resist   b) Refusal
c) Dispel   d) Arrogant

489. Concede
a) Surrender   b) Astute
c) Determined   d) Insistent

490. Compulsory
a) Shower   b) Arid
c) Citadel   d) Mandatory

491. Composure
a) Equilibrium   b) Facet
c) Gutty   d) Loud

492. Compliant
a) Associate   b) Angry
c) Cutting   d) Obedient

493. Complacent
a) Satisfied   b) Clothes
c) Deadly   d) Resist

494. Compelling
a) Shower   b) Aide
c) Clothes   d) Irresistible

495. Commiserate
a) Sympathise   b) Emphasise
c) Dispel   d) Inhuman

496. Commence
a) Resist   b) Refusal
c) Sufficient   d) Initiate

497. Colossal
a) Enormous   b) Puzzle
c) Ample   d) Deadly

498. Collusion
a) Complicated   b) Approval
c) Rise   d) Conspiracy

499. Colloquial
a) Informal   b) Unmoored
c) Sanctuary   d) Cease

500. Cognizant
a) Awe   b) Quit
c) Lessen   d) Aware

501. Conflate
a) Merge   b) caustic
c) Antipathy   d) Eager

502. Confluence
a) Loud   b) Detest
c) Cutting   d) Junction

503. Confound
a) Bewilder   b) Despise
c) Facet   d) Gutty

504. Conglomerate
a) Reliable   b) Avidity
c) Repay   d) Composite

505. Conjecture
a) Speculation   b) Facet
c) Belittle   d) Debase

506. Dally
a) Opaque   b) Angry
c) Cutting   d) Dawdle

507. Dapper
a) Stylish   b) Resist
c) Humanitarian d) Enigmatic

508. Dauntless
a) Charitable   b) Clothes
c) Deadly   d) Bold

509. Dawdle
a) Delay   b) Highlight
c) Emphasize   d) Dispel

510. Dearth
a) Insinuate   b) Detached
c) Distant   d) Scarcity

511. Debacle
a) Catastrophe   b) Unmoored
c) Sanctuary   d) Cease

512. Debilitate
a) Complicated   b) Approval
c) Rise   d) Weaken

513. Debunk
a) Disprove   b) Faithfulness
c) Ease   d) Allay

514. Deduce
a) Despise   b) Facet
c) Gutty   d) Deduct

515. Defame
a) Malign   b) Avidity
c) Repay   d) Adherence

516. Defiance
a) Charge   b) Recount
c) Reliable   d) Disobedience

517. Defunct
a) Extinct   b) Loud
c) Detest   d) Separate

518. Dejected
a) Repay   b) Disaffect
c) Gutty   d) Depressed

519. Deluge
a) Downpour   b) Eagerness
c) Reliable   d) Avidity

520. Denounce
a) Alter   b) Quick
c) Alertness   d) Criticise

521. Depict
a) Describe   b) Rapid
c) Prophet   d) Stern

522. Deplete
a) Belittle   b) Debase
c) Reliable   d) Reduce

523. Derivation
a) Source   b) Calamity
c) Moneyed   d) Upscale

524. Desolate
a) Bottomless   b) Dignified
c) Astonish   d) Lonely

525. Destitute
a) Poor   b) Prophet
c) Stern   d) Alter

526. Deter
a) Creative   b) Affection
c) Sympathy   d) Prevent

527. Detrimental
a) Adverse   b) Announce
c) Disturb   d) Heighten

528. Devout
a) Exhausting   b) Bottomless
c) Artistic   d) Faithful

529. Dexterity
a) Mastery   b) Pleasant
c) Amiable   d) Aid

530. Diabolical
a) Original
b) Fervent
c) Assistance
d) Vile

531. Diatribe
a) Criticism
b) Endless
c) Backing
d) Help

532. Dichotomy
a) Mishap
b) Scam
c) Abstinent
d) Division

533. Diffident
a) Hesitant
b) Stern
c) Alter
d) Calamity

534. Dilettante
a) Disturb
b) Heighten
c) Prophet
d) Ameteurish

535. Dire
a) Critical
b) Desire
c) Pay
d) Announce

536. Enigma
a) Dignified
b) Astonish
c) Shock
d) Mystery

537. Eager
a) Enthusiastic
b) Aid
c) Exhausting
d) Bottomless

538. Emphatic
a) Complex
b) Complicated
c) Approval
d) Pronounced

539. Embellish
a) Decorate
b) Puzzle
c) Ample
d) Deadly

540. Endearing
a) Sufficient
b) Highlight
c) Emphasize
d) Lovable

541. Envelope
a) Cover
b) Inhuman
c) Shower
d) Aide

542. Entice
a) Deadly
b) Resist
c) Associate
d) Attract

543. Enduring
a) Lasting
b) Cutting
c) Facet
d) Gutty

544. Engage
a) Keen
b) Shower
c) Arid
d) Employ

545. Entrap
a) Capture
b) Astute
c) Determined
d) Insistent

546. Fascinate
a) Refusal
b) Dispel
c) Comply
d) Captivate

547. Fasten
a) Attach
b) Unmoored
c) Sanctuary
d) Heed

548. Froth
a) Berate
b) Dispel
c) Inhuman
d) Lather

549. Haughty
a) Arrogant
b) Shower
c) Arid
d) Citadel

550. Hasty
a) Adept
b) Clever
c) Facet
d) Careless

551. Heave
a) Lift
b) Loud
c) Applause
d) Antipathy

552. Hasten
a) Eager
b) Awe
c) Flattery
d) Accelerate

553. Intrigue
a) Mystery
b) Disease
c) Bottomless
d) Dignified

554. Ingenious
a) Rapid
b) Prophet
c) Stern
d) Clever

555. Prototype
a) Model
b) Mystify
c) Harmful
d) Flinch

556. Fierce
a) Grateful   b) Befit
c) Criticise   d) Zealous

557. Painful
a) Punishing   b) Dumbfound
c) Deceive   d) Beast

558. Patrician
a) Blast   b) Desolate
c) Fortress   d) Elite

559. Expedient
a) Device   b) Boycott
c) Dismiss   d) Cruel

560. Abstaining
a) Mystify   b) Harmful
c) Flinch   d) Disciplined

561. Crave
a) Yearn   b) Home
c) Distinction   d) Climb

562. Answer
a) Admiration   b) Curtail
c) Afloat   d) Apologise

563. Display
a) Testify   b) Vindicate
c) Distaste   d) Voracious

564. Garb
a) Stringent   b) Accurate
c) Frugality   d) Costume

565. Quality
a) Trait   b) Deafening
c) Develop   d) Herald

566. Undaunted
a) Apparel   b) Aspect
c) Foolhardy   d) Cheeky

567. Clear
a) Distinct   b) Awe
c) Flattery   d) Authenticate

568. Compound
a) Applause   b) Antipathy
c) Eager   d) Progress

569. Seer
a) Forecast   b) Facet
c) Gutty   d) Loud

570. Harsh
a) Grace   b) Adept
c) Clever   d) Rigid

571. Credible
a) Convincing   b) Shower
c) Arid   d) Citadel

572. Greediness
a) Advert   b) Unmoored
c) Sanctuary   d) Thrift

573. Punish
a) Requite   b) Cease
c) Insinuate   d) Detached

574. Allergy
a) Distant   b) Highlight
c) Emphasise   d) Hatred

575. Ardent
a) Ravenous   b) Dispel
c) Charitable   d) Clothes

576. Esteem
a) Deadly   b) Resist
c) Humanitarian   d) Wonder

577. Abbreviate
a) Downsise   b) Enigmatic
c) Opaque   d) Angry

578. Loose
a) Cutting   b) Facet
c) Belittle   d) Drifting

579. Domicile
a) Address   b) Debase
c) Reliable   d) Avidity

580. Badge
a) Bottomless   b) Dignified
c) Astonish   d) Honor

581. Lift
a) Mounting   b) Shock
c) Desire   d) Pay

582. Stun
 a) Announce   b) Disturb
 c) Heighten   d) Bewilder

583. Evil
 a) Sinister   b) Prophet
 c) Stern   d) Alter

584. Recoil
 a) Calamity   b) Mishap
 c) Scam   d) Refuse

585. Stoppage
 a) Prohibition   b) Abstinent
 c) Endless   d) Backing

586. Exile
 a) Help   b) Original
 c) Fervent   d) Deport

587. Rough
 a) Boorish   b) Assistance
 c) Pleasant   d) Amiable

588. Hail
 a) Aid   b) Exhausting
 c) Bottomless   d) Storm

589. Empty
 a) Desert   b) Artistic
 c) Announce   d) Disturb

590. Stronghold
 a) Heighten   b) Creative
 c) Affection   d) Support

591. Puzzle
 a) Distract   b) Sympathy
 c) Prophet   d) Stern

592. Mislead
 a) Dignified   b) Astonish
 c) Calamity   d) Betray

593. Huge
 a) Mammoth   b) Upscale
 c) Belittle   d) Debase

594. Bound
 a) Reliable   b) Rapid
 c) Prophet   d) Obligated

595. Suit
 a) Ask   b) Stern
 c) Alter   d) Quick

596. Smear
 a) Eagerness   b) Reliable
 c) Avidity   d) Deride

597. Bellicose
 a) Hostile   b) Repay
 c) Disaffect   d) Gutty

598. Mourn
 a) Separate   b) Charge
 c) Recount   d) Rue

599. Preoccupied
 a) Dreamy   b) Avidity
 c) Repay   d) Adherence

600. Kind
 a) Complicated   b) Approval
 c) Rise   d) Favourable

601. Generous
 a) Humanitarian   b) Home
 c) Distinction   d) Climb

602. Castigate
 a) Admiration   b) Curtail
 c) Afloat   d) Scorch

603. Ask
 a) Invoke   b) Vindicate
 c) Distaste   d) Voracious

604. Stain
 a) Stringent   b) Accurate
 c) Frugality   d) Defile

605. Confer
 a) Donate   b) Deafening
 c) Develop   d) Herald

606. Bigotry
 a) Apparel   b) Aspect
 c) Foolhardy   d) Leaning

607. Fight
 a) Tiff   b) Awe
 c) Flattery   d) Authenticate

608. Ramify
a) Applause   b) Antipathy
c) Eager   d) Branch

609. Reciprocal
a) Two-sided   b) Adept
c) Clever   d) Facet

610. Roll
a) Arid   b) Citadel
c) Grace   d) Bloat

611. Bender
a) Heed   b) Advise
c) Berate   d) Drunk

612. Dull
a) Insipid   b) Dispel
c) Inhuman   d) Shower

613. Trumpet
a) Comply   b) Lessen
c) Unmoored   d) Clang

614. Abuse
a) Swearing   b) Resist
c) Refusal   d) Dispel

615. Chilly
a) Astute   b) Determined
c) Insistent   d) Stripped

616. Barefaced
a) Pronounced   b) Shower
c) Arid   d) Citadel

617. Noisy
a) Associate   b) Angry
c) Cutting   d) Clinking

618. Misadventure
a) Mishap   b) Clothes
c) Deadly   d) Resist

619. Naïve
a) Inhuman   b) Shower
c) Aide   d) Infant

620. Bluff
a) Equal   b) Highlight
c) Emphasize   d) Dispel

621. Concede
a) Resist   b) Refusal
c) Sufficient   d) Defer

622. Mutable
a) Fickle   b) Puzzle
c) Ample   d) Deadly

623. Drub
a) Complex   b) Complicated
c) Approval   d) Reprimand

624. Biting
a) Pungent   b) Lessen
c) Unmoored   d) Sanctuary

625. Refrain
a) Eager   b) Awe
c) Quit   d) Finish

626. Dismay
a) Irritation   b) Cutting
c) caustic   d) Antipathy

627. Allure
a) Avidity   b) Repay
c) Despise   d) Magnetism

628. Punish
a) Baste   b) Belittle
c) Debase   d) Reliable

629. Habitual
a) Opaque   b) Angry
c) Cutting   d) Enduring

630. Cagey
a) Safe   b) Resist
c) Humanitarian d) Enigmatic

631. Sneaky
a) Charitable   b) Clothes
c) Deadly   d) Hidden

632. Mercy
a) Charity   b) Highlight
c) Emphasise   d) Dispel

633. Bunch
a) Insinuate   b) Detached
c) Distant   d) Circle

634. Threat
a) Intimidation   b) Unmoored
c) Sanctuary   d) Cease

635. Strong
a) Ease   b) Allay
c) Complicated   d) Forceful

636. Awake
a) Alive   b) Avidity
c) Repay   d) Adherence

637. Atone
a) Exhausting   b) Bottomless
c) Dignified   d) Redeem

638. Attest
a) Authenticate   b) Shock
c) Desire   d) Pay

639. Attire
a) Announce   b) Disturb
c) Heighten   d) Apparel

640. Attribute
a) Aspect   b) Stern
c) Alter   d) Calamity

641. Audacious
a) Mishap   b) Scam
c) Abstinent   d) Foolhardy

642. Audible
a) Deafening   b) Endless
c) Backing   d) Help

643. Augment
a) Original   b) Fervent
c) Assistance   d) Develop

644. Augur
a) Herald   b) Pleasant
c) Amiable   d) Aid

645. Austere
a) Exhausting   b) Bottomless
c) Artistic   d) Stringent

646. Authentic
a) Accurate   b) Announce
c) Disturb   d) Heighten

647. Avarice
a) Creative   b) Affection
c) Sympathy   d) Frugality

648. Avenge
a) Vindicate   b) Prophet
c) Stern   d) Alter

649. Aversion
a) Bottomless   b) Dignified
c) Astonish   d) Distaste

650. Avid
a) Voracious   b) Calamity
c) Moneyed   d) Upscale

651. Awe
a) Debase   b) Reliable
c) Rapid   d) Admiration

652. Abridge
a) Curtail   b) Prophet
c) Stern   d) Alter

653. Adrift
a) Quick   b) Alertness
c) Eagerness   d) Afloat

654. Abode
a) Home   b) Reliable
c) Avidity   d) Repay

655. Ascent
a) Detest   b) Separate
c) Charge   d) Climb

656. Baffle
a) Mystify   b) Recount
c) Reliable   d) Avidity

657. Baleful
a) Repay   b) Adherence
c) Despise   d) Harmful

658. Balk
a) Flinch   b) Faithfulness
c) Ease   d) Allay

659. Ban
a) Complicated   b) Approval
c) Rise   d) Boycott

660. Banish
a) Dismiss   b) Unmoored
c) Sanctuary   d) Cease

661. Barbaric
a) Insinuate   b) Detached
c) Distant   d) Cruel

662. Barrage
a) Blast   b) Emphasize
c) Dispel   d) Charitable

663. Barren
a) Clothes   b) Deadly
c) Resist   d) Desolate

664. Bastion
a) Fortress   b) Humanitarian
c) Enigmatic   d) Opaque

665. Befuddle
a) Angry   b) Cutting
c) Facet   d) Dumbfound

666. Beguile
a) Deceive   b) Belittle
c) Debase   d) Reliable

667. Behemoth
a) Avidity   b) Repay
c) Despise   d) Beast

668. Beholden
a) Grateful   b) Unmoored
c) Sanctuary   d) Cease

669. Behoove
a) Beast   b) Grateful
c) Befit   d) Befit

700. Cacophonous
a) Discordant   b) Fortress
c) Dumbfound   d) Deceive

701. Callow
a) Cruel   b) Blast
c) Desolate   d) Inexperienced

702. Scourge
a) Misadventure   b) Flinch
c) Boycott   d) Dismiss

703. Jellybean
a) Home   b) Distinction
c) Climb   d) Naïve

704. Forthright
a) Bluff   b) Admiration
c) Curtail   d) Afloat

705. Bow
a) Vindicate   b) Distaste
c) Voracious   d) Concede

706. Unstable
a) Mutable   b) Stringent
c) Accurate   d) Frugality

707. Rebuke
a) Deafening   b) Develop
c) Herald   d) Drub

708. Acerbic
a) Biting   b) Apparel
c) Aspect   d) Foolhardy

709. Halt
a) Awe   b) Flattery
c) Authenticate   d) Refrain

710. Drop
a) Concede   b) Heed
c) Advise   d) Berate

711. Crushing
a) Dispel   b) Inhuman
c) Shower   d) Dismay

712. Dazzle
a) Allure   b) Keen
c) Shower   d) Arid

713. Lash
a) Determined   b) Insistent
c) Resist   d) Punish

714. Incurable
a) Habitual   b) Rise
c) Puzzle   d) Ample

715. Vigilant
a) Deadly   b) Resist
c) Refusal   d) Cagey

716. Foxy
a) Sneaky   b) Sufficient
c) Highlight   d) Emphasise

717. Forbearance
a) Dispel   b) Inhuman
c) Shower   d) Mercy

718. Mafia
a) Bunch   b) Aide
c) Clothes   d) Deadly

719. Constraint
a) Lessen   b) Unmoored
c) Sanctuary   d) Threat

720. Shrink
a) Reduce   b) Charitable
c) Clothes   d) Deadly

721. Sick
a) Resist   b) Humanitarian
c) Enigmatic   d) Ailing

722. Simple
a) Uncomplicated   b) Opaque
c) Angry   d) Cutting

723. Singular
a) Facet   b) Belittle
c) Debase   d) Unique

725. Sink
a) Drown   b) Reliable
c) Avidity   d) Repay

726. Slim
a) Despise   b) Facet
c) Gutty   d) Lean

727. Vacant
a) Empty   b) Loud
c) Detest   d) Cutting

728. Vanish
a) Antipathy   b) Eager
c) Awe   d) Disappear

729. Vast
a) Large   b) Quit
c) Lessen   d) Unmoored

730. Victory
a) Complicated   b) Approval
c) Rise   d) Success

731. Virtue
a) Integrity   b) Puzzle
c) Ample   d) Deadly

732. Visible
a) Resist   b) Refusal
c) Sufficient   d) Apparent

734. War
a) Conflict   b) Highlight
c) Emphasize   d) Dispel

735. Wax
a) Resist   b) Associate
c) Angry   d) Grow

736. Weak
a) Feeble   b) Astute
c) Determined   d) Insistent

737. Wet
a) Refusal   b) Dispel
c) Comply   d) Damp

738. White
a) Bleached   b) Lessen
c) Unmoored   d) Sanctuary

739. Wide
a) Heed   b) Advise
c) Berate   d) Broad

740. Win
a) Triumph   b) Dispel
c) Inhuman   d) Shower

741. Wisdom
a) Beautify   b) Shower
c) Arid   d) Knowledge

742. Sweltering
a) Humid   b) Citadel
c) Grace   d) Adept

743. Tall
a) Astonish   b) Shock
c) Desire   d) Towering

744. Tame
a) Docile   b) Announce
c) Disturb   d) Heighten

745. Thick
a) Abstinent   b) Endless
c) Backing   d) Bulky

746. Tight
a) Close   b) Fervent
c) Assistance   d) Pleasant

747. Tiny
a) Amiable   b) Aid
c) Exhausting   d) Small

748. Together
a) Composed   b) Bottomless
c) Artistic   d) Announce

749. Top
a) Prophet   b) Stern
c) Alter   d) Highest

750. Tough
a) Strong   b) Diseased
c) Bottomless   d) Dignified

ANSWERS

SYNONYMS

1. d) Obese	2. a) Misappropriate	3. d) Short
4. a) Opening	5. c) Dignified	6. c) Clever
7. d) Watchful	8. a) Soldier	9. a) Misfortune
10. b) Far	11. b) Imitation	12. c) Accuse
13. c) Rigorous	14. a) Complain	15. b) Paused
16. b) Help	17. a) Try	18. c) Contest
19. b) Rash	20. c) Drunken	21. b) Results
22. d) Betterment	23. d) Sarcastic	24. c) Shifting
25. b) Miserable	26. a) Barren	27. d) Shy
28. b) Free	29. a) Unbiased	30. b) Superficial
31. a) Amusement	32. b) Bankrupt	33. b) Unaccountable
34. a) Weak	35. b) Fleeting	36. a) Uncovered
37. d) Cancel	38. c) Indecency	39. c) Enraptured
40. d) Reprimand	41. d) Hard-working	42. d) Devout
43. c) Examine	44. d) Sometimes	45. c) Obstacle
46. b) Worship	47. c) Forerunner	48. a) Place
49. c) Frank	50. b) Merge	51. a) Hang
52. c) Harassment	53. c) Plenty	54. c) Whole
55. c) Poverty	56. a) Poor	57. b) Frighten
58. a) Quarrelsome	59. c) Complain	60. a) Clown
61. d) Reserve	62. d) Slaughter	63. d) Knowledge
64. b) Vigilant	65. a) Mob	66. c) Excitement
67. a) Think	68. b) Lover of art	69. c) Tremble
70. c) name	71. c) Strict	72. b) Sleeplessness
73. c) Praise	74. d) Reaction	75. a) Offhand
76. d) Economy	77. d) Letters	78. b) Grow
79. a) Excitement	80. c) Summary	81. b) Show up
82. a) Strength	83. c) Adorn	84. b) False
85. c) Loquaciousness	86. b) Gloomy	87. b) Gluttonous
88. d) Waken	89. c) Indulge	90. c) Perilous
91. a) Dishonour	92. a) Crafty	93. b) Glittering
94. b) Warm	95. b) Greedy	96. c) Combine
97. d) Fight	98. d) Dining room	99. a) Ungraceful
100. d) Blunder	101. b) Proportionate	102. d) Disgrace
103. d) Relevant	104. c) Different	105. a) Keep
106. a) Sorrows	107. a) Unsatisfiable	108. b) Lively
109. b) Unconventional	110. d) Deadly	111. d) Unfeeling
112. a) Progress	113. a) Forged	114. a) easily perceived
115. c) Error	116. a) Poor	117. a) Later
118. a) Inventors	119. a) natural tendency	120. d) Optimistic
121. d) Opposed	122. d) Outmanoeuvred	123. a) Compulsory
124. c) Friendship	125. b) Unusual	126. c) Slander
127. b) Exactly	128. c) Absurd	129. b) Suffering

130. d) Intoxicated
131. a) Irrational
132. c) Obscure
133. a) Mutually destructive
134. b) Unruly
135. a) Believable
136. d) Surroundings
137. a) Talks a lot
138. c) Deviation
139. b) Deplorable
140. a) Break
141. a) Complete change
142. c) Unsuspecting
143. a) Rational
144. d) Violence
145. a) Recover
146. a) Foreign
147. d) Dangerous
148. c) Watchful
149. c) Recently
150. b) Non-existent
151. b) Moderated
152. d) Trustworthiness
153. b) Imminent
154. a) Alleviate
155. b) Illegitimate
156. d) Convert
157. c) Vivid
158. b) testaments
159. a) Infer
160. a) Beaten up
161. a) Adjust
162. a) Disinterest
163. b) Strength
164. b) Praised
165. a) Profitable
166. b) Kindness
167. a) Judgment
168. c) Profitable
169. b) Inflamed
170. b) Clear
171. c) Flatterers
172. b) Beginning
173. a) Imitate
174. b) Unmindful
175. d) Unreal
176. c) Uneasiness
177. a) Confirmed
178. b) Pretty
179. b) Whimsical
180. b) Failed
181. a) Entangled
182. a) Defeated
183. c) Rumour
184. d) Diligent
185. b) Obstinate
186. d) Instantaneous
187. d) Humiliated
188. b) Profitable
189. a) Libertine
190. b) Approval
191. d) Sporty
192. d) Privileges
193. b) Fought back
194. c) Lucid
195. c) Destroyed
196. d) Admirable
197. b) hate for women
198. b) Undifferentiated
199. d) Listlessness
200. d) Identification
201. a) very thin
202. d) Abridge
203. a) Unfit for human consumption
204. b) Gentle
205. b) Puzzling
206. b) Show respect and reverance
207. c) Manly
208. c) Disaster
209. c) Homesick
210. c) Occasional
211. a) Wealthy
212. b) Overdramatic
213. d) One appointed by two parties to settle a dispute
214. d) Of the nature of teaching
215. c) Stick used in conducting an orchestra
216. d) Light-hearted
217. c) Pure
218. b) Very stylish
219. a) Wise saying
220. b) Substantiate
221. d) Excited
222. a) Immoral
223. b) waste
224. a) Indirect
225. d) Exempt
226. d) Perfect
227. c) Word formed from abbreviation
228. a) Knowledge
229. a) No longer in existence
230. c) Contradictory
231. b) Repeat
232. d) Yield
233. b) stop doing
234. a) False
235. a) Hiding place
236. a) Few or little
237. b) Hard

238. c) Delight	239. c) Precise	240. c) Pouring forth
241. c) Set free	242. b) Puzzling	243. a) Conditionality
244. b) Greedy	245. d) Praising	246. a) Unsuccessful
247. c) Imitate	248. c) Sudden overthrow of a government	249. b) One that clings
250. b) Quote	251. c) Hungry	252. b) Skill
253. a) Generous	254. b) Initial	255. c) Temporary
256. a) Based on supposition	257. a) Blot out	258. d) Reminding one
259. c) public shame	260. a) mark with spot	261. b) Secretive
262. d) Sacred	263. c) Gather bit by bit	264. d) Merry
265. a) Abuse	266. c) Hesitatingly	267. b) Sleepy
268. a) Beginning	269. a) Trick	270. a) Skeptical
271. c) Outlet for strong emotion	272. a) Unknown	273. d) Discordant
274. d) Rift	275. b) Regret	276. c) Nerve
277. a) Empty boasting	278. c) Like an ox	279. b) Mournful
280. a) Creature	281. a) Having more than one wife or husband	282. c) A great number
283. a) Quibble	284. c) Centre of attraction	285. d) Light shade
286. d) Front of a building	287. a) Inflict	288. c) Honour
289. c) Warmly	290. b) Bright	291. c) Many
292. b) Dispute	293. c) Favouring	294. b) Large
295. c) Vulgar	296. c) Story	297. b) Likely
298. a) Warm	299. a) Dripping	300. b) At once
301. d) Teach	302. d) Tired	303. b) Climate
304. a) Weak	305. a) far	306. c) Modesty
307. b) Stopped	308. a) Likely	309. a) Severe
310. c) Faithful	311. b) Charming	312. a) Regal
313. b) Free	314. a) Missing	315. d) Correct
316. a) Allow	317. a) Living	318. a) Friend
319. d) Old	320. a) Separate	321. d) Ignited
322. c) Confront	323. a) Modify	324. d) Skilled
325. d) Intelligent	326. a) Wretched	327. b) Delay
328. c) Concord	329. c) Confront	330. c) Decide
331. d) Liberate	332. d) Accommodate	333. a) Connect
334. d) Affirm	335. d) Poise	336. d) Welcome
337. a) Confirm	338. a) Kidnap	339. a) Wisdom
340. a) Hurting	341. a) Bewilder	342. a) Pinnacle
343. a) Stern	344. d) Reliable	345. a) Thrift
346. d) Repay	347. a) Hatred	348. d) Ravenous
349. a) Esteem	350. a) Esteem	351. d) Downsize
352. a) Drifting	353. d) Domicile	354. a) Honor

355. d) Mounting	356. a) Puzzle	357. d) Deadly
358. a) Recoil	359. d) Prohibition	360. a) Deport
361. d) Inhuman	362. a) Storm	363. d) Empty
364. a) Help	365. d) Endless	366. a) Shock
367. d) Alter	368. a) Debase	369. d) Detest
370. a) caustic	371. d) Cease	372. a) Complicated
373. d) Sufficient	374. a) Emphasize	375. d) Associate
376. a) Cutting	377. d) Astute	378. a) Insistent
379. d) Heed	380. a) Berate	381. d) Grace
382. a) Clever	383. d) Flattery	384. a) Mishap
385. d) Assistance	386. a) Amiable	387. d) Creative
388. a) Sympathy	389. d) Calamity	390. a) Upscale
391. d) Quick	392. a) Eagerness	393. d) Separate
394. a) Recount	395. d) Faithfulness	396. a) Allay
397. d) Insinuate	398. a) Distant	399. d) Humanitarian
400. a) Opaque	401. a) Uncertain	402. d) Lovable
403. a) Polite	404. d) Spacious	405. a) Bitterness
406. d) Decimate	407. a) Deviation	408. d) Unacknowledged
409. a) Await	410. d) Distaste	411. a) Unconcern
412. d) Leaning	413. a) Capricious	414. d) Mystic
415. a) Old-fashioned	416. d) Original	417. a) Fervent
418. d) Exhausting	419. a) Dignified	420. d) Scam
421. a) Scourge	422. d) Jellybean	423. a) Forthright
424. d) Bow	425. a) Unstable	426. d) Rebuke
427. a) Acerbic	428. d) Halt	429. a) Drop
430. d) Crushing	431. a) Dazzle	432. d) Lash
433. a) Incurable	434. d) Vigilant	435. a) Foxy
436. d) Forbearance	437. a) Mafia	438. d) Constraint
439. a) Compelling	440. d) Conscious	441. a) Maintain
442. d) Poise	443. a) Acquire	444. d) Assert
445. a) Snatch	446. d) Brilliance	447. a) Nagging
448. d) Impress	449. a) Culmination	450. d) Guidance
451. a) Boundless	452. d) Confuse	453. a) Interest
454. d) Degrade	455. a) Scorn	456. d) Nasty
457. a) Cease	458. d) Ideal	459. a) Sufficient
460. d) Underscore	461. a) Aggressive	462. d) Deplore
463. a) Distracted	464. d) Benevolent	465. a) Caring
466. d) Reproach	467. a) Implore	468. d) Lavish
469. a) Penchant	470. d) Disagree	471. a) Divide
472. d) Mutual	473. a) Undulate	474. d) Orgy
475. a) Banal	476. d) Bark	477. a) Heresy
478. d) Cold	479. a) Outright	480. d) Compelling
481. a) Imprison	482. d) Simultaneous	483. a) Forgive

484. d) Harmony	485. a) Gathering	486. d) Brief
487. a) Centred	488. d) Arrogant	489. a) Surrender
490. d) Mandatory	491. a) Equilibrium	492. d) Obedient
493. a) Satisfied	494. d) Irresistible	495. a) Sympathize
496. d) Initiate	497. a) Enormous	498. d) Conspiracy
499. a) Informal	500. d) Aware	501. a) Merge
502. d) Junction	503. a) Bewilder	504. d) Composite
505. a) Speculation	506. d) Dawdle	507. a) Stylish
508. d) Bold	509. a) Delay	510. d) Scarcity
511. a) Catastrophe	512. d) Weaken	513. a) Disprove
514. d) Deduct	515. a) Malign	516. d) Disobedience
517. a) Extinct	518. d) Depressed	519. a) Downpour
520. d) Criticize	521. a) Describe	522. d) Reduce
523. a) Source	524. d) Lonely	525. a) Poor
526. d) Prevent	527. a) Adverse	528. d) Faithful
529. a) Mastery	530. d) Vile	531. a) Criticism
532. d) Division	533. a) Hesitant	534. d) Ameteurish
535. a) Critical	536. d) Mystery	537. a) Enthusiastic
538. d) Pronounced	539. a) Decorate	540. d) Lovable
541. a) Cover	542. d) Attract	543. a) Lasting
544. d) Employ	545. a) Capture	546. d) Captivate
547. a) Attach	548. d) Lather	549. a) Arrogant
550. d) Careless	551. a) Lift	552. d) Accelerate
553. a) Mystery	554. d) Clever	555. a) Model
556. d) Zealous	557. a) Punishing	558. d) Elite
559. a) Device	560. d) Disciplined	561. a) Yearn
562. d) Apologize	563. a) Testify	564. d) Costume
565. a) Trait	566. d) Cheeky	567. a) Distinct
568. d) Progress	569. a) Forecast	570. d) Rigid
571. a) Convincing	572. d) Thrift	573. a) Requite
574. d) Hatred	575. a) Ravenous	576. d) Wonder
577. a) Downsize	578. d) Drifting	579. a) Address
580. d) Honor	581. a) Mounting	582. d) Bewilder
583. a) Sinister	584. d) Refuse	585. a) Prohibition
586. d) Deport	587. a) Boorish	588. d) Storm
589. a) Desert	590. d) Support	591. a) Distract
592. d) Betray	593. a) Mammoth	594. d) Obligated
595. a) Ask	596. d) Deride	597. a) Hostile
598. d) Rue	599. a) Dreamy	600. d) Favourable
601. a) Humanitarian	602. d) Scorch	603. a) Invoke
604. d) Defile	605. a) Donate	606. d) Leaning
607. a) Tiff	608. d) Branch	609. a) Two-sided
610. d) Bloat	611. d) Drunk	612. a) Insipid

613. d) Clang
614. a) Swearing
615. d) Stripped
616. a) Pronounced
617. d) Clinking
618. a) Mishap
619. d) Infant
620. a) Equal
621. d) Defer
622. a) Fickle
623. d) Reprimand
624. a) Pungent
625. d) Finish
626. a) Irritation
627. d) Magnetism
628. a) Baste
629. d) Enduring
630. a) Safe
631. d) Hidden
632. a) Charity
633. d) Circle
634. a) Intimidation
635. d) Forceful
636. a) Alive
637. d) Redeem
638. a) Authenticate
639. d) Apparel
640. a) Aspect
641. d) Foolhardy
642. a) Deafening
643. d) Develop
644. a) Herald
645. d) Stringent
646. a) Accurate
647. d) Frugality
648. a) Vindicate
649. d) Distaste
650. a) Voracious
651. d) Admiration
652. a) Curtail
653. d) Afloat
654. a) Home
655. d) Climb
656. a) Mystify
657. d) Harmful
658. a) Flinch
659. d) Boycott
660. a) Dismiss
661. d) Cruel
662. a) Blast
663. d) Desolate
664. a) Fortress
665. d) Dumbfound
666. a) Deceive
667. d) Beast
668. a) Grateful
669. d) Befit
700. a) Discordant
701. d) Inexperienced
702. a) Misadventure
703. d) Naïve
704. a) Bluff
705. d) Concede
706. a) Mutable
707. d) Drub
708. a) Biting
709. d) Refrain
710. a) Concede
711. d) Dismay
712. a) Allure
713. d) Punish
714. a) Habitual
715. d) Cagey
716. a) Sneaky
717. d) Mercy
718. a) Bunch
719. d) Threat
720. a) Reduce
721. d) Ailing
722. a) Uncomplicated
723. d) Unique
725. a) Drown
726. d) Lean
727. a) Empty
728. d) Disappear
729. a) Large
730. d) Success
731. a) Integrity
732. d) Apparent
734. a) Conflict
735. d) Grow
736. a) Feeble
737. d) Damp
738. a) Bleached
739. d) Broad
740. a) Triumph
741. d) Knowledge
742. a) Humid
743. d) Towering
744. a) Docile
745. d) Bulky
746. a) Close
747. d) Small
748. a) Composed
749. d) Highest
750. a) Strong

MULTIPLE CHOICE QUESTIONS

ANTONYMS

Choose the correct Antonym or Opposite of the given Word from the options provided below in each case.

1) Accept
a) Followed b) Provided
c) Noted d) Rejected

2) Anger
a) Party b) Love
c) Happiness d) Approval

3) Loved
a) Refused b) Hated
c) Defamed d) Averted

4) Obey
a) Attract b) Disobey
c) Repel d) Diffuse

5) Outwit
a) Laugh b) Defeat
c) Victory d) Win

6) Wealthy
a) Wicked b) Famous
c) Poor d) Ill

7) Dull
a) Pale b) Wise
c) Shining d) Colourful

8) Alleviation
a) Lessening b) Magnification
c) Intensify d) Aggravation

9) Receded
a) Bloomed b) Advanced
c) increased d) diminished

10) Transparent
a) Translucent b) Vague
c) Blind d) Opaque

11) Extrovert
a) Introvert b) Boaster
c) Mixer d) Social

12) Virtuous
a) Vicious b) Vulgar
c) Miserly d) Insincere

13) Urban
a) Rustic b) Rural
c) Civil d) Domestic

14) Genuine
a) Bogus b) Rotten
c) Impure d) Unsound

15) Militant
a) Spiritual b) Religious
c) Pacifist d) Combative

16) Unruly
a) Curious b) Obedient
c) Intelligent d) Indifferent

17) Ruthless
a) Militant b) Majestic
c) Might d) Merciful

18) Erudite
a) Ignorant b) Unknown
c) Illiterate d) Unfamiliar

19) Churlish
a) Young b) Cowardly
c) Cultured d) Accommodating

20) Latent
a) Forbidding b) Hidden
c) Obvious d) Artificial

21) Antipathy
a) Indifference b) Fondness
c) Willingness d) Liking

22) Instill
a) Extract b) Expand
c) Express d) Eradicate

23) Eulogistic
a) Brief b) Critical
c) Pretty d) Stern

24) Euphoria
a) Significant b) Literary
c) Strident d) Lethargy

25) Fiasco
a) Success   b) Pollution
c) Mansion   d) Gamble

26) Abundant
a) Infertile   b) Scarce
c) Harsh   d) Prolific

27) Isolation
a) Hardness   b) Segregation
c) Seclusion   d) Association

28) Antiquity
a) Youthfulness b) Recent
c) Common   d) Innovation

29) Hypothesis
a) Theory   b) Fact
c) Conclusive d) Suppressed

30) Parallelism
a) Contrast   b) Disparity
c) Obliquity   d) Divergence

31) Hybrid
a) Composite   b) Familiar
c) Purebred   d) Ignorant

32) Pursue
a) Abandon   b) Discontinue
c) Restrain   d) Deter

33) Diligent
a) Confident   b) Hardworking
c) Lazy   d) Shy

34) Steadfast
a) Staunch   b) Feeble
c) Faint   d) Wavering

35) Conceited
a) Proud   b) Honest
c) Modest   d) Modern

36) Deterrent
a) Determinant b) Detriment
c) Encouragement d) Enrichment

37) Spurious
a) Truthful   b) Authentic
c) Credible   d) Original

38) Deviate
a) Obliviate   b) Break
c) Locate   d) Follow

39) Morose
a) Healthy   b) Gloomy
c) Haggard   d) Cheerful

40) Inspired
a) Overwhelmed b) Dispirited
c) Disillusioned d) Skeptical

41) Autonomous
a) Magnanimous b) Ambiguous
c) Exiguous   d) Dependent

42) Extravagant
a) Developing b) Wonderful
c) Disappearing d) Economical

43) Debonair
a) Awkward   b) Windy
c) Balmy   d) Stomy

44) Exhilarate
a) Gladden   b) Invigorate
c) Shabbily   d) Depress

45) Facsimile
a) Reproduction b) Sincere
c) Original   d) Engineered

46) Fluster
a) Upset   b) Disconcert
c) Confident   d) Disobey

47) Glossy
a) Sleek   b) Ventilating
c) Dull   d) Obscene

48) Ingenuity
a) Skillfulness b) Cunning
c) Sentimental d) Dullness

49) Malign
a) Disparage   b) Slander
c) Praise   d) Purify

50) Swear
a) Support   b) Reject
c) Deny   d) Praise

51) Extrovert
a) Boaster   b) Mixer
c) Introvert   d) Social

52) Ponderous
a) Simple   b) Empty
c) Light   d) Thoughtless

53) Sophisticated
a) Civil   b) Rural
c) Rustic   d) Domestic

54) Avidity
a) Stupidity   b) Greedy
c) Carelessness   d) Overactive

55) Annularity
a) Stubborn   b) Revival
c) Occasionally   d) Smooth

56) Synchronised
a) Adorned   b) Noisy
c) Discordant   d) Following

57) Immaculate
a) Admit   b) Renew
c) Untidy   d) Entertain

58) Inflexible
a) Tender   b) Yielding
c) Soft   d) Tender

59) Rectitude
a) Atheism   b) Smoothness
c) Firmness   d) Deception

60) Dogmatic
a) Simple   b) Spellbound
c) Uncertain   d) Peremptory

61) Progress
a) Reversion   b) Advance
c) Movement   d) Silence

62) Inquisitive
a) Uninterested   b) Dull
c) Careful   d) Indolent

63) Fabulous
a) Real   b) Poor
c) Literary   d) Commonplace

64) Erratic
a) Right   b) Punctual
c) Free   d) Reliable

65) Considerable
a) Usual   b) Common
c) Inadequate   d) Inattentive

66) Cynical
a) Crazy   b) Naive
c) Mature   d) Eccentric

67) Objective
a) Personal   b) Subjective
c) Deleted   d) Intimate

68) Mitigate
a) Repair   b) Worsen
c) Expedite   d) Slacken

69) Brilliant
a) Shining   b) Dull
c) Flat   d) Apparent

70) Retrogressive
a) Advancing   b) Progressive
c) Forwarding   d) Improving

71) Bridge
a) Release   b) Open
c) Bind   d) Divide

72) Deleterious
a) Vital   b) Nourishing
c) Fatal   d) Injurious

73) Strident
a) stable   b) Pleasant
c) Musical   d) Melodious

74) Relinquish
a) Persist   b) Claim
c) Stick to   d) Possess

75) Nostalgic
a) Airy   b) Ambitious
c) Forgetful   d) Wistful

76) Heterogeneous
a) Similar   b) different
c) Colourful   d) Homogeneous

77) Candid
a) Taciturn b) Frank
c) Close d) Silent

78) Flamboyant
a) Angry b) Excited
c) Quiet d) Exclaimed

79) Austerity
a) Extreme b) Harsh
c) Ascetic d) Lenience

80) Turbulence
a) Noisy b) Calmness
c) Hostility d) Impropriety

81) Peer
a) Equal b) Equivalent
c) Certain d) Unequal

82) Haggard
a) Shrewed b) Plump
c) Vast d) Maidenly

83) Dank
a) Babbling b) Gutters
c) Wet d) Dry

84) Churlish
a) Modest b) Coarse
c) Naughty d) Courteous

85) Fantastic
a) Real b) Wonderful
c) Economical d) Illusion

86) Derogatory
a) Roguish b) Praising
c) immediate d) Conferred

87) Prim
a) Private b) Prior
c) Formal d) Informal

88) Deferential
a) Respectful b) Disrespectful
c) Disorganised d) Distinguishable

89) Outstrip
a) Cover b) Follow
c) Cooperate d) Compete

90) Compliant
a) Adamant b) Elementary
c) Defective d) Appreciative

91) Autonomy
a) Submissiveness b) Dependence
c) Subordination d) Slavery

92) Shallow
a) High b) Deep
c) Hidden d) Hollow

93) Overt
a) Deep b) Shallow
c) Secret d) unwritten

94) Accord
a) Solution b) Act
c) Dissent d) Concord

95) Alive
a) Passive b) Dead
c) Asleep d) Drowsy

96) Synthetic
a) Cosmetic b) Plastic
c) Affable d) Natural

97) Precarious
a) Dangerous b) Cautious
c) Safe d) Easy

98) Deep
a) Elementary b) Shallow
c) Superficial d) Perfunctory

99) Lend
a) Hire b) Pawn
c) Cheat d) Borrow

100) Paucity
a) Surplus b) Scarcity
c) Presence d) Richness

101) Minor
a) Heavy b) Tall
c) Major d) Big

102) Appropriate
a) Unskilled b) Unsuitable
c) Unqualified d) Unable

103) Opaque
a) Misty
b) Covered
c) Clear
d) Transparent

104) Ruthless
a) Mindful
b) Compassionate
c) Majestic
d) Merciful

105) Violent
a) Tame
b) Humble
c) Gentle
d) Harmless

106) Dearth
a) Extravagance
b) Scarcity
c) Abundance
d) Sufficiency

107) Up
a) Coloured
b) Childlike
c) Down
d) Imminent

108) Exhibit
a) Conceal
b) Prevent
c) Withdraw
d) Concede

109) Haughty
a) Pitiable
b) Scared
c) Humble
d) Cowardly

110) Virtue
a) Vice
b) Fraud
c) Wickedness
d) Crime

111) Erudite
a) Professional
b) Immature
c) Unimaginative
d) Ignorant

112) Acquitted
a) Entrusted
b) Convicted
c) Burdened
d) Freed

113) Laconic
a) Prolix
b) Profligate
c) Prolific
d) Bucolic

114) Absolute
a) Scarce
b) Limited
c) Faulty
d) Deficient

115) Magnify
a) Induce
b) Diminish
c) Destroy
d) Shrink

116) Enormous
a) Soft
b) Tiny
c) Average
d) Weak

117) Commissioned
a) Started
b) Finished
c) Closed
d) Terminated

118) Artificial
a) Red
b) Truthful
c) Natural
d) Solid

119) Exodus
a) Influx
b) Return
c) Homecoming
d) restoration

120) Relinquish
a) Abdicate
b) Possess
c) Renounce
d) Deny

121) Expand
a) Convert
b) Congest
c) Condense
d) Conclude

122) Mortal
a) Divine
b) Spiritual
c) Immortal
d) Eternal

123) Quiescent
a) Active
b) Weak
c) Dormant
d) Unconcerned

124) Obeying
a) Ordering
b) Refusing
c) Following
d) Contradicting

125) Fraudulent
a) Candid
b) Forthright
c) Direct
d) Genuine

126) Flagitious
a) Candid
b) Forthright
c) Direct
d) Genuine

127) Belittle
a) Criticise
b) Exaggerate
c) Flatter
d) Adore

128) Startled
a) Amused
b) Endless
c) Relaxed
d) Astonished

129) Busy
a) Occupied   b) Relaxed
c) Engrossed   d) Engaged

130) Fresh
a) Faulty   b) Disgraceful
c) Sluggish   d) Stale

131) Culpable
a) Defendable   b) Careless
c) Blameless   d) Irresponsible

132) Evasive
a) Free   b) Liberal
c) Honest   d) Frank

133) Gregarious
a) Antisocial   b) Horrendous
c) Glorious   d) Similar

134) Aware
a) Uncertain   b) Sure
c) Ignorant   d) Doubtful

135) Hirsute
a) Scaly   b) Erudite
c) Bald   d) Quiet

136) Shrink
a) Contract   b) Expand
c) Spoil   d) Stretch

137) Common
a) Rare   b) Petty
c) Small   d) Poor

138) Comfort
a) Uncomfort   b) Discomfort
c) Miscomfort   d) Ease

139) Dear
a) Priceless   b) Worthless
c) Free   d) Cheap

140) Arrogant
a) Humble   b) Egotistic
c) Cowardly   d) Gentlemanly

141) Victorious
a) Defeated   b) Destroyed
c) Annexed   d) Vanquished

142) Graceful
a) Rough   b) Miserable
c) Expert   d) Awkward

143) Nadir
a) Modernity   b) Liberty
c) Zenith   d) Progress

144) Extravagance
a) Luxury   b) Economical
c) Poverty   d) Cheapness

145) Pertinent
a) Irrational   b) Insistent
c) Irregular   d) Irrelevant

146) Obscure
a) Implicit   b) Explicit
c) Obnoxious   d) Pedantic

147) Urbane
a) Illiterate   b) Discourteous
c) Backward   d) Orthodox

148) Vanity
a) Pride   b) Conceit
c) Humility   d) Ostentatious

149) Rarely
a) Hardly   b) Frequently
c) definitely   d) Periodically

150) Malicious
a) Kind   b) Generous
c) Boastful   d) Indifferent

151) Epilogue
a) Dialogue   b) Postscript
c) Prelude   d) Epigram

152) Capacious
a) Limited   b) Foolish
c) Caring   d) Changeable

153) Condense
a) Expand   b) Interpret
c) Distribute   d) Lengthen

154) Adaptable
a) Adoptable   b) Yielding
c) Flexible   d) Rigid

155) Sacrosanct
a) Irreligious   b) Irreverent
c) Unethical   d) Unholy

156) Indiscreet
a) Reliable   b) Prudent
c) Honest   d) Stupid

157) Familiar
a) Unpleasant   b) Friendly
c) Dangerous   d) Strange

158) Tangible
a) Ethereal   b) Actual
c) Concrete   d) Solid

159) Love
a) Villainy   b) Compulsion
c) Hatred   d) Force

160) Famous
a) Disgraced   b) Evil
c) Unknown   d) Popular

161) Absolute
a) Deficient   b) Limited
c) Faulty   d) Scarce

162) Frugal
a) Copious   b) Generous
c) Extravagant   d) Ostentatious

163) Insipid
a) Tasty   b) Discreet
c) Stupid   d) Feast

164) Able
a) Disable   b) Unable
c) Inable   d) Misable

165) Hostility
a) Courtesy   b) Relationship
c) Hospitality   d) Friendliness

166) Crowded
a) Busy   b) Quiet
c) Congested   d) Deserted

167) Comic
a) Emotional   b) Fearful
c) Tragic   d) Painful

168) Hapless
a) Cheerful   b) Fortunate
c) Consistent   d) Shapely

169) Flimsy
a) Frail   b) Firm
c) Filthy   d) Flippant

170) Equanimity
a) Resentment   b) Duplicity
c) Dubiousness   d) Excitement

171) Addition
a) Division   b) Subtraction
c) Enumeration   d) Multiplication

172) Zenith
a) Acme   b) Nadir
c) Top   d) Pinnacle

173) Doubtful
a) Famous   b) Fixed
c) Certain   d) Important

174) Perrenial
a) Frequent   b) Lasting
c) Regular   d) Rare

175) Benign
a) Malevolent   b) friendly
c) Soft   d) Unwise

176) Hindrance
a) Aid   b) Cooperation
c) Persuasion   d) Agreement

177) Extricate
a) Manifest   b) Release
c) Palpable   d) Entangle

178) Repress
a) Inhibit   b) Curb
c) Liberate   d) Quell

179) Acquitted
a) Freed   b) Convicted
c) Burdened   d) Entrusted

180) Provocation
a) Vocation   b) Peace
c) Pacification   d) Destruction

181) Subservient
a) Aggresive   b) Dignified
c) Straightforward d) Supercilious

182) Lend
a) Borrow   b) Pawn
c) Cheat   d) Hire

183) Faint-hearted
a) Warm-hearted b) Hot-blooded
c) Full-blooded d) Stout-hearted

184) Remiss
a) Forgetful   b) Dutiful
c) Watchful   d) Harmful

185) Vacant
a) Semi-transparent b) Occupied
c) Muddy   d) dark

186) Honorary
a) Dishonorable b) Paid
c) Reputed   d) Official

187) Meticulous
a) Mutual   b) Meretricious
c) Shaggy   d) Slovenly

188) Loquacious
a) Reticent   b) Garrulous
c) Talkative   d) Verbose

189) Confess
a) deny   b) Contest
c) Refuse   d) Contend

190) Annoy
a) Praise   b) Please
c) Rejoice   d) Reward

191) Repel
a) Attend   b) Continue
c) Concentrate d) Attract

192) Suppress
a) Encourage   b) Praise
c) Allow   d) Permit

193) Niggardly
a) Frugal   b) Stingy
c) Thrifty   d) Generous

194) Impasse
a) Resurgence b) Continuation
c) Breakthrough d) Combination

195) Haphazard
a) Fortuitous   b) deliberate
c) Indifferent   d) Accidental

196) Density
a) Rarity   b) Clarity
c) Intelligence   d) Brightness

197) Adherent
a) Detractor   b) Alien
c) Enemy   d) Rival

198) Base
a) Climax   b) Top
c) Height   d) Roof

199) Patchy
a) Attractive   b) Simple
c) Uniform   d) Clear

200) Enmity
a) Important   b) Friendship
c) Unnecessary d) Likeness

201) Hollow
a) Filled   b) Strong
c) Solid   d) Substantial

202) Valuable
a) Invaluable   b) Inferior
c) Worthless   d) Lowly

203) Gullible
a) Incredulous b) Easy
c) Smart   d) Stylish

204) Industrious
a) Indifferent   b) casual
c) Indolent   d) Passive

205) Autonomy
a) Slavery   b) Dependence
c) Subordination d) Submissiveness

206) Alien
a) Native   b) Natural
c) Domiciled   d) Resident

207) Synthetic
a) Affable   b) Plastic
c) Natural   d) Cosmetic

208) Balance
a) Disbalance   b) Debalance
c) Misbalance   d) Imbalance

209) Liability
a) Property   b) Debt
c) Assets   d) Treasure

210) Mountain
a) Plain   b) Precipice
c) Plateau   d) Valley

211) Stationary
a) Active   b) Rapid
c) Mobile   d) Busy

212) Concede
a) Object   b) Grant
c) Refuse   d) Accede

213) Violent
a) Humble   b) Gentle
c) Harmless   d) Tame

214) Virtuous
a) Wicked   b) Vicious
c) Corrupt   d) Scandalous

215) Gain
a) Loose   b) Lost
c) Fall   d) Lose

216) Preliminary
a) Final   b) Secondary
c) First   d) Initial

217) Defiance
a) Anxiety   b) Suspicion
c) Obedience   d) Dismay

218) Encourage
a) Dampen   b) Discourage
c) Disapprove   d) Warn

219) Lucid
a) Glory   b) Obscure
c) Noisy   d) Distinct

220) Stringent
a) General   b) Lenient
c) Vehement   d) Magnanimous

221) Minor
a) Big   b) Tall
c) Major   d) Heavy

222) Revealed
a) Denied   b) Ignored
c) Concealed   d) Overlooked

223) Essential
a) Extra   b) Minors
c) Noughts   d) Trivial

224) Hypocritical
a) Gentle   b) Amiable
c) Sincere   d) Dependable

225) Fickle
a) Courageous   b) Steadfast
c) Sincere   d) Humble

226) Abounds
a) Shines   b) Suffices
c) Lacks   d) Fails

227) Barbarians
a) Civilized   b) Uncivilized
c) Cruel   d) Bad

228) Feasible
a) Impractical b) Difficult
c) Impossible   d) Impracticable

229) Crestfallen
a) Vainglorious b) Triumphant
c) Indignant   d) Disturbed

230) Feasibility
a) Unsuitability b) Impropriety
c) Cheapness   d) Impracticality

231) Incessant
a) Intermittent b) Soft
c) Harsh   d) Constant

232) Exodus
a) Invasion   b) Immigration
c) Entry   d) Expulsion

233) Resist
  a) Fight   b) Welcome
  c) Accept   d) Repel

234) Superfluous
  a) Important   b) Significant
  c) Relevant   d) Essential

235) Reluctant
  a) Wanting   b) Anxious
  c) Willing   d) Eager

236) Impertinent
  a) Healthy   b) Adequate
  c) Respectful   d) Smooth

237) Comprehensive
  a) Casual   b) Indifferent
  c) Inadequate   d) Superficial

238) Impracticable
  a) Easy   b) Feasible
  c) Possible   d) Alternate

239) Asset
  a) Loss   b) Drag
  c) Liability   d) Handicap

240) Humility
  a) Pride   b) Arrogance
  c) Insolence   d) Conceit

241) Collision
  a) Retaliatory   b) Conciliatory
  c) Perfunctory d) Circuitous

242) Elation
  a) Despondency b) Disappointment
  c) Misery   d) Despair

243) Expedite
  a) Postpone   b) Adjourn
  c) Defer   d) delay

244) Intelligent
  a) Dull   b) Ignorant
  c) Weak   d) Simple

245) Abhor
  a) Admire   b) Applaud
  c) Respect   d) Appreciate

246) Insipid
  a) Lively   b) Loud
  c) Argumentative d) Curious

247) Squandering
  a) Discarding   b) Collecting
  c) Boarding   d) Saving

248) Rear
  a) Unusual   b) Upper
  c) Front   d) Back

249) Overt
  a) Converse   b) Covert
  c) Pervert   d) Contrived

250) Zeal
  a) Indifference b) Despair
  c) Calmness   d) Passiveness

251) Progressive
  a) Revolutionary b) Brave
  c) Retrograde   d) Outmoded

252) Effeminacy
  a) Aggresiveness b) Manliness
  c) Attractiveness d) Boorishness

253) Adversity
  a) Sincerity   b) Curiosity
  c) Animosity   d) Prosperity

254) Improvised
  a) Complete   b) Permanent
  c) Preplanned   d) proscribed

255) Initiated
  a) Confused   b) Started
  c) Closed   d) Compliacted

256) Delectable
  a) Heavy   b) Tasty
  c) Unsavoury   d) Nice

257) Morbid
  a) Healthy   b) Insipid
  c) Cheerful   d) Appealing

258) Pragmatic
  a) Indefinite   b) Idealistic
  c) Vague   d) Optimistic

259) Levity
a) Seriousness   b) Religiosity
c) Solemnity   d) Gravity

260) Memorable
a) Passing   b) Forgetful
c) Immemorial   d) Innocuous

261) Humility
a) Grandeur   b) Friendliness
c) Arrogance   d) Decency

262) Enthusiasm
a) Eagerness   b) Indifference
c) Weakness   d) Softness

263) Stiff
a) Courteous   b) Soft
c) Flexible   d) Lively

264) Haphazard
a) Planned   b) Extraordinary
c) Excellent   d) Designed

265) Abandoned
a) Supported   b) Pleased
c) Encouraged   d) Saved

266) Obscurity
a) Clarity   b) Definiteness
c) Precision   d) Specificity

267) Progressive
a) Regressive   b) Retrograde
c) Obstructive   d) Abhorrent

268) Corpulent
a) Fat   b) Garrulous
c) Belligerent   d) gaunt

269) Vindictive
a) Forgetful   b) Obedient
c) Forgiving   d) Timid

270) Precipitate
a) Aggravate   b) defer
c) Create   d) Push

271) Ambiguity
a) Clarity   b) Rationality
c) Certainty   d) Perversity

272) Material
a) Internal   b) Psychic
c) Spiritual   d) Celestial

273) Ominous
a) Pleasant   b) Auspicious
c) Encouraging   d) Favourable

274) Affluence
a) Indigence   b) Sorrow
c) Opulence   d) Poverty

275) Congenial
a) Disagreeable   b) Unpleasant
c) Inconvenient   d) Unsuitable

276) Meager
a) Continuous   b) hard
c) Fabulous   d) Adequate

277) Applauded
a) Dissaproved   b) Praised
c) Misunderstood   d) Welcomed

278) Following
a) Succeeding   b) Preceding
c) Proceeding   d) Receding

279) Superficial
a) Mysterious   b) Profound
c) Difficult   d) Mystical

280) Rebuked
a) Received   b) Invited
c) Awarded   d) Praised

281) Pernicious
a) Permanent   b) Parochial
c) Beneficial   d) Dangerous

282) Accelerate
a) Supervise   b) Control
c) Slacken   d) Check

283) Massive
a) Meagre   b) Light
c) Heavy   d) Short

284) Prudent
a) Shortsighted   b) Inconsiderate
c) Reckless   d) Injudicious

285) **Magnanimity**
   a) Enmity
   b) Jealousy
   c) Meanness
   d) Poverty

286) **Inevitable**
   a) Inevident
   b) Ineligible
   c) Inefficient
   d) Uncertain

287) **Confirms**
   a) Strengthens
   b) Contradicts
   c) Opposes
   d) Verifies

288) **Humility**
   a) Pride
   b) Honesty
   c) Determination
   d) Gentleness

289) **Tactful**
   a) Disciplined
   b) Strict
   c) Naive
   d) Tactless

290) **Incidental**
   a) Intentional
   b) Usual
   c) Conventional
   d) Permissible

291) **Dilapidated**
   a) Neglected
   b) Renovated
   c) Regenerated
   d) Furnished

292) **Friendly**
   a) Helpful
   b) Quiet
   c) Understanding
   d) Hostile

293) **Ostentation**
   a) Miserliness
   b) Purity
   c) Simplicity
   d) Innocence

294) **Disparage**
   a) Please
   b) belittle
   c) Praise
   d) Denigrate

295) **Amused**
   a) Frightened
   b) Astonished
   c) Jolted
   d) Saddened

296) **Absence**
   a) Above
   b) Untidy
   c) Presence
   d) Wise

297) **Abundant**
   a) Wide
   b) Accidental
   c) Wrong
   d) Scarce

298) **Accept**
   a) Wet
   b) Worst
   c) Refuse
   d) Help

299) **Accurate**
   a) Anti-clockwise
   b) Wise
   c) Worse
   d) Inaccurate

300) **Admit**
   a) Deny
   b) Appear
   c) Wealth
   d) Without

301) **Advance**
   a) Weak
   b) Retreat
   c) Wise
   d) Attic

302) **Advantage**
   a) Waste
   b) Wild
   c) Awake
   d) Disadvantage

303) **Agree**
   a) Beginning
   b) Wide
   c) Ward
   d) Disagree

304) **Alive**
   a) Wet
   b) Borrower
   c) War
   d) Dead

305) **Ally**
   a) West
   b) Enemy
   c) Wane
   d) Bottom

306) **Always**
   a) Wealth
   b) Never
   c) Deny
   d) Calm

307) **Ancient**
   a) Departure
   b) Weak
   c) Captivity
   d) Modern

308) **Answer**
   a) Waste
   b) Depth
   c) Cheerful
   d) Question

309) **Approached**
   a) Departed
   b) Descend
   c) Ward
   d) Cheerful

310) **Approval**
   a) Destroy
   b) War
   c) Child
   d) Disapproval

311) Arrival
   a) Difficult   b) Wane
   c) Bright   d) Departure

312) Artificial
   a) Disadvantage b) natural
   c) CLient   d) Vice

313) Ascend
   a) Cloudy   b) Disagree
   c) Vertical   d) Descend

314) Asleep
   a) Valueless   b) Awake
   c) Disapproval   d) Clumsy

315) Attack
   a) Valley   b) Collect
   c) Discomfort   d) defense

316) Attention
   a) Inattention   b) Discourage
   c) Complicated   d) Cloudy

317) Attractive
   a) Repulsive   b) Compulsory
   c) Rude   d) Lie

318) Backward
   a) Dishonest   b) Consonant
   c) Forward   d) Untidy

319) Bad
   a) Good   b) Contract
   c) Dislike   d) Unsightly

320) beautiful
   a) Ugly   b) Coward
   c) Disloyal   d) Unsatisfactory

321) Beginning
   a) Disobedient   b) Qualified
   c) Ending   d) Cowardice

322) Below
   a) Displease   b) Coward
   c) Unlikely   d) Above

323) Bend
   a) Unlawful   b) Straighten
   c) Crooked   d) Distant

324) Best
   a) Worst   b) Distribute
   c) Unknown   d) Cry

325) Better
   a) Worse   b) Collect
   c) Curse   d) Dull

326) Big
   a) Complicated   b) Small
   c) Customer   d) Stupid

327) Bitter
   a) Compulsory   b) Uninhabited
   c) Sweet   d) Heavy

328) Blame
   a) Praise   b) Diseased
   c) Dawdle   d) Consonant

329) Bless
   a) Dawn   b) Curse
   c) Unfortunate   d) Contract

330) Blunt
   a) Day   b) Sharp
   c) Unfold   d) Coward

331) Bold
   a) Timid   b) Understand
   c) Cowardice   d) Dead

332) Borrow
   a) Lend   b) Dear
   c) Ruthless   d) Ugly

333) Bravery
   a) Cowardice   b) Troubled
   c) Decrease   d) Crooked

334) Bright
   a) Trivial   b) Defeat
   c) Dull   d) In

335) Broad
   a) Defense   b) Inaccurate
   c) Minute   d) Narrow

336) Build
   a) Inattention   b) Demagnetize
   c) Meek   d) destroy

337) Calm
a) Troubled   b) Thirst
c) Deny   d) Incapable

338) Capable
a) Incorrect   b) Incapable
c) Thin   d) departure

339) Captivity
a) Thin   b) Increase
c) Depth   d) Liberty

400) Careful
a) careless   b) Indefinite
c) Descend   d) Stout

401) Cellar
a) There   b) demolish
c) Attic   d) Energetic

402) Cheap
a) Expensive   b) Lie
c) tenant   d) Difficult

403) Clear
a) Disadvantage   b) lend
c) Cloudy   d) Temporary

404) Clever
a) Disagree   b) late
c) Stupid   d) Sweet

405) Clockwise
a) Disapproval   b) Anti-clockwise
c) Sweet   d) Last

406) Close
a) Discomfort   b) Distant
c) Supply   d) Big

407) Cold
a) Superior   b) Hot
c) Discourage   d) Kind

408) Combine
a) separate   b) Succeed
c) Joy   d) Rude

409) Come
a) Go   b) Subject
c) Dishonest   d) Irregularly

410) Comfort
a) Discomfort   b) Rude
c) Powerful   d) Unlike

411) Common
a) Rare   b) Disloyal
c) Stupid   d) Dishonest

412) Conceal
a) Dislike   b) reveal
c) Disobedient   d) Student

413) Correct
a) Incorrect   b) Straighten
c) Disloyal   d) Displease

414) Courage
a) Stale   b) Distant
c) Disobedient   d) Cowardice

415) Courteous
a) Distribute   b) Displease
c) Rude   d) Spendthrift

416) Cruel
a) Distant   b) Down
c) Kind   d) South

417) Cunning
a) Sorry   b) Simple
c) free   d) drunk

418) Dainty
a) Clumsy   b) Dull
c) Soft   d) Liberty

419) Danger
a) Soft   b) Safety
c) Dwarf   d) Full

420) Dark
a) Light   b) Genuine
c) Employee   d) Smooth

421) Decrease
a) Empty   b) Increase
c) Small   d) Give

422) Deep
a) Shallow   b) Slow
c) Encourage   d) Go

423) **Definite**
 a) Ending
 b) Slow
 c) Good
 d) Indefinite

424) **Demand**
 a) Enemy
 b) Harmless
 c) Loose
 d) Supply

425) **Despair**
 a) Hope
 b) Liberty
 c) Simple
 d) Enemy

426) **Disappear**
 a) Appear
 b) Full
 c) Even
 d) Shut

427) **Discourage**
 a) Exclude
 b) Shorten
 c) genuine
 d) Encourage

428) **Disease**
 a) Health
 b) Give
 c) Exhale
 d) Short

429) **Dismal**
 a) Exit
 b) Go
 c) Short
 d) Cheerful

430) **Doctor**
 a) Sharp
 b) Good
 c) Patient
 d) Outside

431) **Dry**
 a) External
 b) Harmless
 c) Shallow
 d) Wet

432) **Dull**
 a) bright
 b) health
 c) Failure
 d) Servant

433) **Dusk**
 a) Separate
 b) Distant
 c) Dawn
 d) High

434) **Early**
 a) feeble
 b) Separate
 c) Hinder
 d) late

435) **East**
 a) West
 b) Find
 c) Hope
 d) senior

436) **Easy**
 a) Host
 b) Difficult
 c) First
 d) Seldom

437) **Ebb**
 a) Hot
 b) secretive
 c) Flow
 d) Glow

438) **Economize**
 a) Sea
 b) Waste
 c) Ignorance
 d) Follower

439) **Employer**
 a) Scarce
 b) Employee
 c) Folly
 d) Liberty

440) **Empty**
 a) Forward
 b) Onward
 c) Full
 d) Careless

441) **Encourage**
 a) sane
 b) Free
 c) Discourage
 d) Attic

442) **End**
 a) Safety
 b) Dear
 c) Beginning
 d) Freedom

443) **Entrance**
 a) Full
 b) Vague
 c) Exit
 d) Sad

444) **Excited**
 a) Stupid
 b) Rush
 c) Calm
 d) genuine

445) **Expand**
 a) Rough
 b) Contract
 c) Give
 d) Take

446) **Expensive**
 a) Go
 b) Right
 c) Cheap
 d) Distant

447) **Export**
 a) Hot
 b) reveal
 c) Good
 d) Import

448) **Exterior**
 a) Harmless
 b) Interior
 c) Retreat
 d) Dishonest

449) External
a) Health   b) Internal
c) Rude   d) Repulsive

450) Fail
a) Remember   b) Succeed
c) Discourage   d) High

451) Famous
a) Unknown   b) Hinder
c) Refused   d) Discomfort

452) Fast
a) Disapproval   b) Refuse
c) Hope   d) Slow

453) Fat
a) Disagree   b) Thin
c) Host   d) Refuse

454) Feeble
a) Hot   b) Sturdy
c) Disadvantage   d) receded

455) Few
a) Difficult   b) Reap
c) Ignorance   d) many

456) Find
a) Immature   b) Lose
c) rare   d) Destroy

457) First
a) Last   b) Impatient
c) Quiet   d) descend

458) Fold
a) Rude   b) Unfold
c) Question   d) depth

459) Foolish
a) Pupil   b) Wise
c) Import   d) Departure

460) Forelegs
a) deny   b) Impossible
c) Public   d) Hind legs

461) Forget
a) Proud   b) demagnetize
c) Imprudent   d) Remember

462) Fortunate
a) Impure   b) Unfortunate
c) Prose   d) defense

463) Found
a) In   b) Lost
c) Defeat   d) Present

464) Frank
a) Presence   b) Inaccurate
c) Secretive   d) Decrease

465) Freedom
a) Inattention   b) Praise
c) rare   d) Captivity

466) Frequent
a) Seldom   b) Reveal
c) Incapable   d) Poor

467) Fresh
a) Incorrect   b) Stale
c) Plural   d) Incorrect

468) Friend
a) Enemy   b) Soft
c) Increase   d) Hull

469) Full
a) Indefinite   b) pessimist
c) Empty   d) Rude

470) Gather
a) Patient   b) Distribute
c) Industrious.   d) Kind

471) Generous
a) Simple   b) Cheap
c) Outside   d) mean

472) Gentle
a) Injustice   b) Rough
c) Opaque   d) Clumsy

473) Giant
a) dwarf   b) Safety
c) Old   d) Innocent

474) Glad
a) Insecurity   b) Sorry
c) Occupied   d) Light

475) Gloomy
a) Increase   b) Nonsense
c) Cheerful   d) Interior

476) Granted
a) Shallow   b) Refused
c) Internal   d) New

477) Great
a) Indefinite   b) Minute
c) Invisible   d) Ordinary

478) Guardian
a) Irregularly   b) Supply
c) natural   d) Ward

479) Guest
a) Joy   b) Host
c) Destroy   d) narrow

480) Guilty
a) Kind   b) Innocent
c) Descend   d) More

481) Happy
a) Depth   b) sad
c) Large   d) Modern

482) Hard
a) Sad   b) Last
c) Departure   d) Soft

483) Harmful
a) Deny   b) Harmless
c) Small   d) Late

484) Hasten
a) Cloudy   b) Dawdle
c) Minimum   d) Lend

485) Hate
a) Love   b) Lie
c) Mean   d) Defense

486) Healthy
a) Light   b) many
c) Defeat   d) Unhealthy

487) Heavy
a) Light   b) Majority
c) Light   d) Decrease

488) Height
a) Lowly   b) Dear
c) Liquid   d) Depth

489) Here
a) Listener   b) There
c) Dead   d) Love

490) Hero
a) Coward   b) Lost
c) day   d) Little

491) Hill
a) Lose   b) Valley
c) Dawn   d) Lost

492) Hinder
a) Lost   b) Dawdle
c) Little   d) Aid

493) Honest
a) Listener   b) Dark
c) Dishonest   d) Love

494) Horizontal
a) Liquid   b) Customer
c) Vertical   d) Lowly

495) Humble
a) Light   b) Proud
c) Curse   d) Majority

496) Hunger
a) Cry   b) Light
c) Thirst   d) Many

497) Imitation
a) Crooked   b) Lie
c) Mean   d) Genuine

498) Immense
a) Tiny   b) Lend
c) Minimum   d) Murky

499) Imprison
a) Caulk   b) Minute
c) Free   d) Late

500) Include
a) Last   b) Mirthless
c) Exclude   d) Dawn

501) Increase
a) Modern   b) Contract
c) Much   d) Decrease

502) Inferior
a) Superior   b) Kind
c) More   d) Consonant

503) Inhabited
a) Uninhabited   b) Narrow
c) Joy   d) Compulsory

504) Inhale
a) Irregularly   b) Complicated
c) Exhale   d) Natural

505) Inside
a) Collect   b) Invisible
c) Outside   d) Never

506) Intelligent
a) Stupid   b) New
c) Internal   d) Clumsy

507) Intentional
a) Accidental   b) Unintentional
c) Cloudy   d) Interior

508) Interesting
a) Occupied   b) Insecurity
c) Client   d) Dull

509) Interior
a) Old   b) Clear
c) Innocent   d) Exterior

510) Internal
a) Opaque   b) Unlawful
c) External   d) Injustice

511) Join
a) Outside   b) Inexpensive
c) Unknown   d) Separate

512) Junior
a) Patient   b) Industrious
c) Dull   d) Senior

513) Justice
a) Indefinite   b) Injustice
c) Stupid   d) Pessimist

514) King
a) Uninhabited   b) Subject
c) Increase   d) Pliable

515) Knowledge
a) Ignorance   b) Incorrect
c) Plural   d) Diseases

516) Land
a) Incapable   b) Poor
c) Sea   d) Unfortunate

517) Landlord
a) Tenant   b) Unfold
c) Inattention   d) Praise

518) Large
a) Presence   b) Inaccurate
c) Small   d) Understand

519) Last
a) In   b) Ugly
c) Present   d) First

520) Laugh
a) Impure   b) Cry
c) Troubled   d) prose

521) Lawful
a) Unlawful   b) Proud
c) Trivial   d) Imprudent

522) Lawyer
a) Tiny   b) Impossible
c) Public   d) Client

523) Lazy
a) Import   b) Timid
c) Energetic   d) Pupil

524) Leader
a) Follower   b) Thirst
c) Query   d) Impolite

525) Lecturer
a) Student   b) Thin
c) Quiet   d) Impatient

526) Left
a) Thin   b) Right
c) rare   d) Immature

527) Lender
a) Borrower b) Reap
c) Stout d) Ignorant

528) Lengthen
a) Shorten b) Hot
c) Receded d) departed

529) Less
a) More b) Tenant
c) Refuse d) Host

530) Light
a) Hope b) Temporary
c) Dark d) Refuse

531) Like
a) Hinder b) Sweet
c) Dislike d) Refused

532) Likely
a) Remember b) Unlikely
c) Sweet d) High

533) Little
a) Large b) health
c) Supply d) Repulsive

534) Lofty
a) Superior b) Lowly
c) harmless d) Retire

535) Long
a) Reveal b) Good
c) Succeed d) Short

536) Loss
a) Go b) Win
c) Subject d) Right

537) Loud
a) Give b) Soft
c) Rough d) Powerful

538) Low
a) High b) Stupid
c) Genuine d) Rush

539) Loyal
a) Sad b) Disloyal
c) Full d) Student

540) Mad
a) Safety b) Sane
c) Freedom d) Straighten

541) Magnetize
a) Sane b) Free
c) Stale d) Demagnetize

542) Master
a) Scarce b) Servant
c) Spendthrift d) Onward

543) Mature
a) South b) Immature
c) Scarce d) Folly

544) Maximum
a) Follower b) Sea
c) Minimum d) Sorry

545) Me
a) Flow b) You
c) Soft d) Secretive

546) Merry
a) First b) Mirthless
c) Seldom d) Soft

547) Minority
a) Smooth b) Majority
c) Senior d) Win

548) Miser
a) Spendthrift b) Small
c) Feeble d) Weak

549) Misunderstand
a) Slow b) separate
c) Understand d) Distant

550) Narrow
a) Servant b) Slow
c) Failure d) Wide

551) Near
a) Slack b) External
c) Shallow d) Far

552) Neat
a) Simple b) Untidy
c) Exterior d) Sharp

553) New
  a) Short   b) Shut
  c) Exit   d) Old

554) Night
  a) Exhale   b) Short
  c) Shorten   d) Day

555) Noisy
  a) Quiet   b) Short
  c) Exclude   d) Shorten

556) North
  a) Short   b) Even
  c) South   d) Open

557) Obedient
  a) Simple   b) Disobedient
  c) Sharp   d) Enemy

558) Odd
  a) Shallow   b) Foster
  c) Slack   d) Even

559) Offer
  a) Ending   b) Slow
  c) Servant   d) Refuse

560) Open
  a) Shut   b) Encourage
  c) Slow   d) Crooked

561) Optimist
  a) Pessimist b) Separate
  c) Empty   d) Little

562) Out
  a) Smooth   b) Senior
  c) Employee d) In

563) Parent
  a) Child   b) Dwarf
  c) Seldom   d) Soft

564) Past
  a) Soft   b) Present
  c) Dull   d) Secretive

565) Patient
  a) Sorry   b) Sea
  c) Impatient d) Drunk

566) Peace
  a) South   b) Down
  c) war   d) Scarce

567) Permanent
  a) Temporary b) Spendthrift
  c) Less   d) Distribute

568) Please
  a) Displease b) Sane
  c) Stale   d) Distant

569) Plentiful
  a) Safety   b) Straighten
  c) Displease d) Lacking

570) Poetry
  a) Prose   b) sad
  c) Disobedient d) Student

571) Polite
  a) Rush   b) Impolite
  c) Disloyal   d) Stupid

572) Possible
  a) Sturdy   b) Dislike
  c) Rough   d) Impossible

573) Poverty
  a) Right   b) Dishonest
  c) Subject   d) Wealth

574) Powerful
  a) Weak   b) Rude
  c) Succeed   d) Reveal

575) Pretty
  a) Discourage b) Retreat
  c) Unsightly d) Superior

576) Private
  a) Supply   b) repulsive
  c) Discomfort d) Public

577) Prudent
  a) Imprudent b) Disapproval
  c) Remember d) Sweet

578) Pure
  a) Impure   b) Disagree
  c) Refused   d) Sweet

579) Qualified
a) Disadvantage   b) refuse
c) Temporary   d) Unqualified

580) Rapid
a) refuse   b) Tenant
c) Difficult   d) Slow

581) Regularly
a) destroy   b) There
c) Irregularly   d) receded

582) Rich
a) Poor   b) Descend
c) Thick   d) reap

583) Right
a) Thin   b) Deep
c) rare   d) Wrong

584) Rigid
a) Departure   b) Thin
c) Pliable   d) Quiet

585) Rough
a) Thirst   b) Question
c) Smooth   d) Deny

586) Satisfactory
a) Unsatisfactory   b) derailed
c) detain   d) Jerk

587) Scatter
a) Public   b) Minute
c) Collect   d) defense

588) Second-hand
a) New   b) defeat
c) Approval   d) trivial

589) Security
a) Insecurity   b) Decrease
c) troubled   d) Disagree

590) Sense
a) Ugly   b) Dear
c) Nonsense   d) Disadvantage

591) Serious
a) Understand   b) trivial
c) Difficult   d) Dead

592) Shopkeeper
a) Unfold   b) Public
c) day   d) Customer

593) Simple
a) Dawn   b) Imprudent
c) Complicated   d) Unfortunate

594) Singular
a) Impure   b) Plural
c) Diseased   d) Unhealthy

595) Slim
a) dark   b) Uninhabited
c) Stout   d) Qualified

596) Sober
a) stupid   b) Drunk
c) Customer   d) Slow

597) Solid
a) Dull   b) Irregularly
c) Curse   d) Liquid

598) Sorrow
a) Unknown   b) cry
c) Joy   d) Poor

599) Sour
a) crooked   b) sweet
c) Wrong   d) left

600) Sow
a) Unlikely   b) reap
c) Soft   d) brave

601)Speaker
a) Cowardice   b) Smooth
c) Listener   d) Unqualified

602) Stand
a) Free   b) Coward
c) Lie   d) Tally

603) Straight
a) Contract   b) Crooked
c) Collect   d) Ugly

604) Strong
a) Untidy   b) new
c) Consonant   d) Weak

605) Success
  a) failure   b) Compulsory
  c) Insecurity   d) Untruth

606) Sunny
  a) Cloudy   b) Vague
  c) Complicated d) Nonsense

607) Take
  a) Give   b) Valley
  c) Trivial   d) Collect

608) Tall
  a) Clumsy   b) Superior
  c) Short   d) valueless

609) Tame
  a) vertical   b) Cloudy
  c) Wild   d) Supply

610) Teacher
  a) Sweet   b) Vice
  c) Pupil   d) Client

611) Thick
  a) Wane   b) bright
  c) sweet   d) Thin

612) Tight
  a) Loose   b) war
  c) Child   d) Temporary

613) Top
  a) Cheerful   b) Bottom
  c) Tenant   d) ward

614) Truth
  a) Waste   b) Cheerful
  c) Lie   d) There

615) Valuable
  a) Valueless   b) Thirst
  c) Borrower   d) wet

616) Victory
  a) Timid   b) Wide
  c) defeat   d) Arsenal

617) Virtue
  a) Awake   b) Vice
  c) Tiny   d) Wild

618) Visible
  a) Trivial   b) Invisible
  c) Attic   d) Wise

619) Voluntary
  a) Appear   b) troubled
  c) Without   d) Compulsory

620) Vowel
  a) Clock   b) Ugly
  c) Worse   d) Consonant

621) Wax
  a) Aid   b) Worst
  c) Understand   d) Wane

622) Wisdom
  a) Unfold   b) Accidental
  c) Folly   d) Wrong

623) Within
  a) Without   b) Above
  c) Unfortunate d) You

624) Frequent
  a) Poor   b) Incapable
  c) Reveal   d) seldom

625) Fresh
  a) Plural   b) Incorrect
  c) Stale   d) Correct

626) Past
  a) Soft   b) Present
  c) Foe   d) deft

627) Full
  a) Pessimist   b) Indefinite
  c) Empty   d) Rude

628) Captivity
  a) Bondage   b) Liberty
  c) Slavery   d) caprice

629) Secretive
  a) Frank   b) Honesty
  c) Polite   d) Rich

630) Adept
  a) Incapable   b) Aid
  c) Exhausting   d) Bottomless

631) Astute
a) Foolish   b) Dignified
c) Astonish   d) Shock

632) Abject
a) Commendable   b) Desire
c) Pay   d) Announce

633) Adjourn
a) Advance   b) Disturb
c) Heighten   d) Prophet

634) Accord
a) Disagreement b) Stern
c) Alter   d) Calamity

635) Accost
a) Ignore   b) Mishap
c) Scam   d) Abstinent

636) Adjudge
a) Defer   b) Endless
c) Backing   d) Help

637) Acquit
a) Accuse   b) Original
c) Fervent   d) Assistance

638) Adjust
a) Disarrange   b) Pleasant
c) Amiable   d) Aid

639) Adjoin
a) Disconnect   b) Exhausting
c) Bottomless   d) Artistic

640) Avouch
a) Abandon   b) Announce
c) Disturb   d) Heighten

641) Aplomb
a) Fear   b) Creative
c) Affection   d) Sympathy

642) Accept
a) Reject   b) Prophet
c) Stern   d) Alter

643) Affirm
a) Deny   b) Disease
c) Bottomless   d) Dignified

644) Abduct
a) Release   b) Astonish
c) Calamity   d) Moneyed

645) Acumen
a) Ignorance   b) Upscale
c) Belittle   d) Debase

646) Aching
a) Healthy   b) Reliable
c) Rapid   d) Prophet

647) Amaze
a) Bore   b) Stern
c) Alter   d) Quick

648) Apex
a) Base   b) Alertness
c) Eagerness   d) Reliable

649) Advice
a) Oppose   b) Repay
c) Disaffect   d) Gutty

650) Affect
a) Dissuade   b) Loud
c) Detest   d) Separate

651) Abase
a) Grow   b) Charge
c) Recount   d) Reliable

652) Abhor
a) Admire   b) Avidity
c) Repay   d) Adherence

653) Abrasive
a) Agreeable   b) Despise
c) Facet   d) Gutty

654) Abstain
a) Embrace   b) Faithfulness
c) Ease   d) Allay

655) Abstract
a) Real   b) Complicated
c) Approval   d) Rise

656) Abundant
a) Needy   b) Advert
c) Unmoored   d) Sanctuary

657) Accentuate
a) Mask   b) Cease
c) Insinuate d) Detached

658) Accomplice
a) Antagonist b) Distant
c) Highlight d) Emphasize

659) Acrimonious
a) Happy   b) Dispel
c) Charitable d) Clothes

660) Acute
a) Blunt   b) Deadly
c) Resist   d) Humanitarian

661) Adamant
a) Flexible   b) Enigmatic
c) Opaque   d) Angry

662) Adhere
a) Disobey   b) Cutting
c) Facet   d) Belittle

663) Admonish
a) Commend   b) Debase
c) Reliable   d) Avidity

664) Adorn
a) Disfigure b) Repay
c) Despise   d) Facet

665) Adroit
a) Awkward   b) Gutty
c) Loud   d) Detest

666) Adulation
a) Abuse   b) Cutting
c) caustic   d) Antipathy

667) Adversity
a) Advantage b) Eager
c) Awe   d) Quit

668) Advocacy
a) Stop   b) Lessen
c) Unmoored   d) Sanctuary

669) Affable
a) Hateful   b) Cease
c) Complex   d) Complicated

670) Affinity
a) Dislike   b) Approval
c) Rise   d) Puzzle

671) Affliction
a) Blessing   b) Ample
c) Deadly   d) Resist

672) Affluent
a) Destitute b) Refusal
c) Sufficient d) Highlight

673) Agile
a) Depressed b) Emphasize
c) Dispel   d) Inhuman

674) Alacrity
a) Apathy   b) Shower
c) Aide   d) Clothes

675) Alienate
a) Combine   b) Deadly
c) Resist   d) Associate

676) Allege
a) Deny   b) Angry
c) Cutting   d) Facet

677) Allegiance
a) Apathy   b) Keen
c) Shower   d) Arid

678) Allude
a) Abstain   b) Citadel
c) Astute   d) Determined

679) Aloof
a) Friendly   b) Insistent
c) Resist   d) Refusal

680) Altruistic
a) Stingy   b) Comply
c) Lessen   d) Unmoored

681) Ambiguous
a) Certain   b) Sanctuary
c) Heed   d) Advise

682) Ambivalent
a) Determined b) Berate
c) Dispel   d) Inhuman

683) Amiable
a) Hostile   b) Beautify
c) Shower   d) Arid

684) Amicable
a) Disagreeable   b) Citadel
c) Grace   d) Adept

685) Ample
a) Cramped   b) Clever
c) Facet   d) Gutty

686) Animosity
a) Like   b) Loud
c) Applause   d) Antipathy

687) Annihilate
a) Establish   b) Eager
c) Awe   d) Flattery

688) Anomaly
a) Conformity   b) Authenticate
c) Apparel   d) Aspect

689) Balk
a) Accept   b) Foolhardy
c) Deafening   d) Develop

690) Ban
a) Approval   b) Herald
c) Stringent   d) Accurate

691) Banish
a) Allow   b) Frugality
c) Vindicate   d) Distaste

692) Barbaric
a) Civilized   b) Voracious
c) Admiration   d) Curtail

693) Barrage
a) Dribble   b) Afloat
c) Home   d) Distinction

694) Barren
a) Fruitful   b) Climb
c) Mystify   d) Harmful

695) Bastion
a) Weakness   b) Dismiss
c) Cruel   d) Blast

696) Befuddle
a) Enlighten   b) Desolate
c) Fortress   d) Dumbfound

697) Beguile
a) Refuse   b) Deceive
c) Beast   d) Grateful

698) Behemoth
a) Lightweight   b) Bottomless
c) Dignified   d) Astonish

699) Beholden
a) Ingrateful   b) Shock
c) Desire   d) Pay

700) Behoove
a) Unsuitable   b) Heighten
c) Prophet   d) Stern

701) Belittle
a) Approve   b) Alter
c) Calamity   d) Mishap

702) Belligerent
a) Agreeable   b) Scam
c) Abstinent   d) Endless

703) Bemoan
a) Praise   b) Backing
c) Help   d) Original

704) Bemused
a) Disinterested   b) Fervent
c) Assistance   d) Pleasant

705) Benign
a) Unfriendly   b) Amiable
c) Aid   d) Exhausting

706) Benevolent
a) Cruel   b) Bottomless
c) Artistic   d) Announce

707) Berate
a) Compliment   b) Disturb
c) Heighten   d) Creative

708) Beseech
a) Answer   b) Affection
c) Sympathy   d) Prophet

709) Besmirch
a) Clean   b) Bottomless
c) Dignified   d) Astonish

710) Bestow
a) Deny   b) Calamity
c) Moneyed   d) Upscale

711) Bias
a) Fairness   b) Belittle
c) Debase   d) Reliable

712) Bicker
a) Agree   b) Rapid
c) Prophet   d) Stern

713) Bifurcate
a) Join   b) Alter
c) Quick   d) Alertness

714) Bilateral
a) Multilateral b) Eagerness
c) Reliable   d) Avidity

715) Billowing
a) Shrink   b) Repay
c) Disaffect   d) Gutty

716) Bland
a) Exciting   b) Loud
c) Detest   d) Separate

717) Blasphemy
a) Respect   b) Charge
c) Recount   d) Reliable

718) Bleak
a) Bright   b) Avidity
c) Repay   d) Adherence

719) Blatant
a) Concealed   b) Despise
c) Facet   d) Gutty

720) Cacophonous
a) Quiet   b) Faithfulness
c) Ease   d) Allay

721) Calamity
a) Creation   b) Complicated
c) Approval   d) Rise

723) Callow
a) Experienced b) Advert
c) Unmoored   d) Sanctuary

724) Candid
a) Biased   b) Cease
c) Insinuate   d) Detached

725) Capitulate
a) Conquer   b) Emphasize
c) Dispel   d) Charitable

726) Capricious
a) Cautious   b) Clothes
c) Deadly   d) Resist

727) Castigate
a) Approve   b) Humanitarian
c) Enigmatic   d) Opaque

728) Caustic
a) Bland   b) Angry
c) Cutting   d) Facet

729) Cease
a) Begin   b) Debase
c) Reliable   d) Avidity

730) Cede
a) Fight   b) Repay
c) Despise   d) Facet

731) Chagrin
a) Confidence b) Loud
c) Detest   d) Cutting

732) Charisma
a) Dull   b) Antipathy
c) Eager   d) Awe

733) Chastise
a) Laud   b) Quit
c) Lessen   d) Unmoored

734) Chronic
a) Halting   b) Sanctuary
c) Cease   d) Complex

735) Circumspect
a) Careless b) Complicated
c) Approval d) Rise

736) Clandestine
a) Forthright b) Puzzle
c) Ample d) Deadly

737) Clemency
a) Meanness b) Resist
c) Refusal d) Sufficient

738) Clique
a) Individual b) Highlight
c) Emphasize d) Dispel

739) Coercion
a) Consent b) Inhuman
c) Shower d) Aide

740) Cogent
a) Vague b) Resist
c) Associate d) Angry

741) Avarice
a) Generosity b) Shower
c) Arid d) Citadel

742) Avenge
a) Forgive b) Astute
c) Determined d) Insistent

743) Aversion
a) Respect b) Resist
c) Refusal d) Dispel

744) Avid
a) Dispassionate b) Comply
c) Lessen d) Unmoored

745) Awe
a) Disregard b) Sanctuary
c) Heed d) Advise

746) Abridge
a) Expand b) Berate
c) Dispel d) Inhuman

747) Adrift
a) Anchored b) Beautify
c) Shower d) Arid

748) Abode
a) Annex b) Citadel
c) Grace d) Adept

749) Accolade
a) Censure b) Antipathy
c) Eager d) Awe

750) Ascent
a) Decline b) Authenticate
c) Apparel d) Aspect

ANSWERS

ANTONYMS

1. d) Rejected
2. d) Approval
3. b) Hated
4. b) Disobey
5. b) Defeat
6. c) Poor
7. c) Shining
8. a) Lessening
9. c) Increased
10. d) Opaque
11. a) Introvert
12. b) Vulgar
13. b) Rural
14. a) Bogus
15. c) Pacifist
16. b) Obedient
17. d) Merciful
18. a) Ignorant
19. c) Cultured
20. c) Obvious
21. d) Liking
22. a) Extract
23. b) Critical
24. d) Lethargy
25. a) Success
26. b) Scarce
27. b) Segregation
28. b) Recent
29. b) Fact
30. a) Contrast
31. c) Purebred
32. a) Abandon
33. c) Lazy
34. d)Wavering
35. c) Modest
36. c) Encouragement
37. b) Authentic
38. d) Follow
39. d) Cheerful
40. b) Dispirited
41. d) Dependent
42. d) Economical
43. a) Awkward
44. d) Depress
45. c) Original
46. c) Confident
47. c) Dull
48. d) Dullness
49. c) Praise
50. d) Praise
51. c) Introvert
52. d) Thoughtless
53. c) Rustic
54. c) Carelessness
55. c) Occasionally
56. c) Discordant
57. c) Untidy
58. b) Yielding
59. d) Deception
60. a) Simple
61. a) Reversion
62. a) Uninterested
63. d) Commonplace
64. d) Reliable
65. c) Inadequate
66. c) Mature
67. b) Subjective
68. b) Worsen
69. b) Dull
70. b) Progressive
71. d) Divide
72. a) Vital
73. d) Melodious
74. b) Claim
75. c) Forgetful
76. d) Homogeneous
77. a) Taciturn
78. c) Quiet
79. d) Lenience
80. b) Calmness
81. d) Unequal
82. d) Maidenly
83. d) Dry
84. a) Modest
85. a) Real
86. b) Praising
87. d) Informal
88. b) Disrespectful
89. a) Cover
90. a) Adamant
91. b) Dependence
92. b) Deep
93. c) Secret
94. c) Dissent
95. b) Dead
96. d) Natural
97. c) Safe
98. b) Shallow
99. d) Borrow
100. a) Surplus
101. c) Major
102. b) Unsuitable
103. d) Transparent
104. b) Compassionate
105. c) Gentle
106. c) Abundance
107. c) Down
108. a) Conceal
109. c) Humble
110. a) Vice
111. d) Ignorant
112. b) Convicted
113. c) Prolific
114. b) Limited
115. d) Shrink
116. b) Tiny
117. d) Terminated
118. c) Natural
119. a) Influx
120. b) Possess
121. c) Condense
122. c) Immortal
123. d) Unconcerned
124. b) Refusing
125. d) Genuine
126. b) Forthright
127. c) Flatter
128. c) Relaxed
129. b) Relaxed

130. d) Stale
131. c) Blameless
132. c) Honest
133. a) Antisocial
134. c) Ignorant
135. c) Bald
136. b) Expand
137. a) Rare
138. b) Discomfort
139. d) Cheap
140. a) Humble
141. a) Defeated
142. d) Awkward
143. c) Zenith
144. b) Economical
145. d) Irrelevant
146. a) Implicit
147. b) Discourteous
148. c) Humility
149. b) Frequently
150. a) Kind
151. c) Prelude
152. a) Limited
153. a) Expand
154. d) Rigid
155. b) Irreverent
156. a) Reliable
157. d) Strange
158. a) Ethereal
159. c) Hatred
160. c) Unknown
161. b) Limited
162. b) Generous
163. a) Tasty
164. b) Unable
165. d) Friendliness
166. d) Deserted
167. c) Tragic
168. c) Consistent
169. b) Firm
170. a) Resentment
171. b) Subtraction
172. b) Nadir
173. c) Certain
174. d) Rare
175. a) Malevolent
176. b) Cooperation
177. d) Entangle
178. c) Liberate
179. b) Convicted
180. c) Pacification
181. d) Supercilious
182. a) Borrow
183. d) Stout-hearted
184. b) Dutiful
185. b) Occupied
186. a) Dishonorable
187. d) Slovenly
188. a) Reticent
189. a) Deny
190. b) Please
191. d) Attract
192. a) Encourage
193. d) Generous
194. c) Breakthrough
195. b) Deliberate
196. a) Rarity
197. a) Detractor
198. b) Top
199. c) Uniform
200. b) Friendship
201. a) Filled
202. c) Worthless
203. c) Smart
204. c) Indolent
205. a) Slavery
206. a) Native
207. c) Natural
208. d) Imbalance
209. c) Assets
210. a) Plain
211. a) Active
212. c) Refuse
213. b) Gentle
214. a) Wicked
215. d) Lose
216. a) Final
217. c) Obedience
218. b) Discourage
219. b) Obscure
220. b) Lenient
221. c) Major
222. c) Concealed
223. d) Trivial
224. c) Sincere
225. b) Steadfast
226. c) Lacks
227. a) Civilized
228. a) Impractical
229. b) Triumphant
230. d) Impracticality
231. a) Intermittent
232. d) Expulsion
233. c) Accept
234. d) Essential
235. c) Willing
236. c) Respectful
237. c) Inadequate
238. b) Feasible
239. c) Liability
240. d) Conceit
241. d) Circuitous
242. a) Despondency
243. d)Delay
244. b) Ignorant
245. a) Admire
246. a) Lively
247. d) Saving
248. c) Front
249. b) Covert
250. d) Passiveness
251. c) Retrograde
252. b) Manliness
253. d) Prosperity
254. a) Complete
255. c) Closed
256. c) Unsavoury
257. c) Cheerful
258. b)Idealistic

259. a) Seriousness	260. b) Forgetful	261. c) Arrogance
262. b) Indifference	263. c) Flexible	264. a) Planned
265. a) Supported	266. a) Clarity	267. a) Regressive
268. d)Gaunt	269. c) Forgiving	270. b)Defer
271. a) Clarity	272. c) Spiritual	273. b) Auspicious
274. d) Poverty	275. b) Unpleasant	276. d) Adequate
277. a) Dissaproved	278. b) Preceding	279. b) Profound
280. d) Praised	281. c) Beneficial	282. d) Check
283. a) Meagre	284. c) Reckless	285. c) Meanness
286. d) Uncertain	287. b) Contradicts	288. a) Pride
289. d) Tactless	290. b) Usual	291. b) Renovated
292. d) Hostile	293. c) Simplicity	294. c) Praise
295. d) Saddened	296. c) Presence	297. d) Scarce
298. c)Refuse	299. d) Inaccurate	300. a) Deny
301. b) Retreat	302. d) Disadvantage	303. d) Disagree
304. d) Dead	305. b) Enemy	306. b) Never
307. d) Modern	308. d) Question	309. a)Departed
310. d) Disapproval	311. d) Departure	312. b)Natural
313. d) Descend	314. b) Awake	315. d)Defense
316. a) Inattention	317. a) Repulsive	318. c) Forward
319. a) Good	320. a) Ugly	321. c) Ending
322. d) Above	323. b) Straighten	324. a) Worst
325. a) Worse	326. b) Small	327. c) Sweet
328. a) Praise	329. b) Curse	330. b) Sharp
331. a) Timid	332. a) Lend	333. a) Cowardice
334. c) Dull	335. d) Narrow	336. d)Destroy
337. a) Troubled	338. b) Incapable	339. d) Liberty
400. a)Careless	401. c) Attic	402. a) Expensive
403. c) Cloudy	404. c) Stupid	405. b) Anti-clockwise
406. b) Distant	407. b) Hot	408. a)Separate
409. a) Go	410. a) Discomfort	411. a) Rare
412. b) Reveal	413. a) Incorrect	414. d) Cowardice
415. c) Rude	416. c) Kind	417. b) Simple
418. a) Clumsy	419. b) Safety	420. a) Light
421. b) Increase	422. a) Shallow	423. d) Indefinite
424. d) Supply	425. a) Hope	426. a) Appear
427. d) Encourage	428. a) Health	429. d) Cheerful
430. c) Patient	431. d) Wet	432. a)Bright
433. c) Dawn	434. d)Late	435. a) West
436. b) Difficult	437. c) Flow	438. b) Waste
439. b) Employee	440. c) Full	441. c) Discourage
442. c) Beginning	443. c) Exit	444. c) Calm
445. b) Contract	446. c) Cheap	447. d) Import

448. b) Interior	449. b) Internal	450. b) Succeed
451. a) Unknown	452. d) Slow	453. b) Thin
454. b) Sturdy	455. d)Many	456. b) Lose
457. a) Last	458. b) Unfold	459. b) Wise
460. d) Hind legs	461. d) Remember	462. b) Unfortunate
463. b) Lost	464. c) Secretive	465. d) Captivity
466. a) Seldom	467. b) Stale	468. a) Enemy
469. c) Empty	470. b) Distribute	471. d)Mean
472. b) Rough	473. a)Dwarf	474. b) Sorry
475. c) Cheerful	476. b) Refused	477. d) Ordinary
478. d) Ward	479. b) Host	480. b) Innocent
481. b)Sad	482. d) Soft	483. b) Harmless
484. b) Dawdle	485. a) Love	486. d) Unhealthy
487. c) Light	488. a) Lowly	489. b) There
490. a) Coward	491. b) Valley	492. d) Aid
493. c) Dishonest	494. c) Vertical	495. b) Proud
496. c) Thirst	497. d) Genuine	498. a) Tiny
499. c) Free	500. c) Exclude	501. d) Decrease
502. a) Superior	503. a) Uninhabited	504. c) Exhale
505. c) Outside	506. a) Stupid	507. b) Unintentional
508. d) Dull	509. d) Exterior	510. c) External
511. d) Separate	512. d) Senior	513. b) Injustice
514. b) Subject	515. a) Ignorance	516. c) Sea
517. a) Tenant	518. c) Small	519. d) First
520. b) Cry	521. a) Unlawful	522. d) Client
523. c) Energetic	524. a) Follower	525. a) Student
526. b) Right	527. a) Borrower	528. a) Shorten
529. a) More	530. c) Dark	531. c) Dislike
532. b) Unlikely	533. a) Large	534. b) Lowly
535. d) Short	536. b) Win	537. b) Soft
538. a) High	539. b) Disloyal	540. b) Sane
541. d) Demagnetize	542. b) Servant	543. b) Immature
544. c) Minimum	545. b) You	546. b) Mirthless
547. b) Majority	548. a) Spendthrift	549. c) Understand
550. d) Wide	551. d) Far	552. b) Untidy
553. d) Old	554. d) Day	555. a) Quiet
556. c) South	557. b) Disobedient	558. d) Even
559. d) Refuse	560. a) Shut	561. a) Pessimist
562. d) In	563. a) Child	564. b) Present
565. c) Impatient	566. c)War	567. a) Temporary
568. a) Displease	569. d) Lacking	570. a) Prose
571. b) Impolite	572. d) Impossible	573. d) Wealth
574. a) Weak	575. c) Unsightly	576. d) Public

577. a) Imprudent

580. d) Slow

583. d) Wrong

586. a) Unsatisfactory

589. a) Insecurity

592. d) Customer

595. c) Stout

598. c) Joy

601. c) Listener

604. d) Weak

607. a) Give

610. c) Pupil

613. b) Bottom

616. c) Defeat

619. d) Compulsory

622. c) Folly

625. c) Stale

628. b) Liberty

631. a) Foolish

634. a) Disagreement

637. a) Accuse

640. a) Abandon

643. a) Deny

646. a) Healthy

649. a) Oppose

652. a) Admire

655. a) Real

658. a) Antagonist

661. a) Flexible

664. a) Disfigure

667. a) Advantage

670. a) Dislike

673. a) Depressed

676. a) Deny

679. a) Friendly

682. a) Determined

685. a) Cramped

688. a) Conformity

691. a) Allow

694. a) Fruitful

697. a) Refuse

700. a) Unsuitable

703. a) Praise

578. a) Impure

581. c) Irregularly

584. c) Pliable

587. c) Collect

590. c) Nonsense

593. c) Complicated

596. b) Drunk

599. b) Sweet

602. c) Lie

605. a) Failure

608. c) Short

611. d) Thin

614. c) Lie

617. b) Vice

620. d) Consonant

623. a) Without

626. b) Present

629. a) Frank

632. a) Commendable

635. a) Ignore

638. a) Disarrange

641. a) Fear

644. a) Release

647. a) Bore

650. a) Dissuade

653. a) Agreeable

656. a) Needy

659. a) Happy

662. a) Disobey

665. a) Awkward

668. a) Stop

671. a) Blessing

674. a) Apathy

677. a) Apathy

680. a) Stingy

683. a) Hostile

686. a) Like

689. a) Accept

692. a) Civilized

695. a) Weakness

698. a) Lightweight

701. a) Approve

704. a) Disinterested

579. d) Unqualified

582. a) Poor

585. c) Smooth

588. a) New

591. b) Trivial

594. b) Plural

597. d) Liquid

600. b) Reap

603. b) Crooked

606. a) Cloudy

609. c) Wild

612. a) Loose

615. a) Valueless

618. b) Invisible

621. d) Wane

624. d) Seldom

627. c) Empty

630. a) Incapable

633. a) Advance

636. a) Defer

639. a) Disconnect

642. a) Reject

645. a) Ignorance

648. a) Base

651. a) Grow

654. a) Embrace

657. a) Mask

660. a) Blunt

663. a) Commend

666. a) Abuse

669. a) Hateful

672. a) Destitute

675. a) Combine

678. a) Abstain

681. a) Certain

684. a) Disagreeable

687. a) Establish

690. a) Approval

693. a) Dribble

696. a) Enlighten

699. a) Ingrateful

702. a) Agreeable

705. a) Unfriendly

706. a) Cruel
707. a) Compliment
708. a) Answer
709. a) Clean
710. a) Deny
711. a) Fairness
712. a) Agree
713. a) Join
714. a) Multilateral
715. a) Shrink
716. a) Exciting
717. a) Respect
718. a) Bright
719. a) Concealed
720. a) Quiet
721. a) Creation
723. a) Experienced
724. a) Biased
725. a) Conquer
726. a) Cautious
727. a) Approve
728. a) Bland
729. a) Begin
730. a) Fight
731. a) Confidence
732. a) Dull
733. a) Laud
734. a) Halting
735. a) Careless
736. a) Forthright
737. a) Meanness
738. a) Individual
739. a) Consent
740. a) Vague
741. a) Generosity
742. a) Forgive
743. a) Respect
744. a) Dispassionate
745. a) Disregard
746. a) Expand
747. a) Anchored
748. a) Annex
749. a) Censure
750. a) Decline

CAREER & BUSINESS MANAGEMENT

CONCISE DICTIONARIES

All books available at www.vspublishers.com

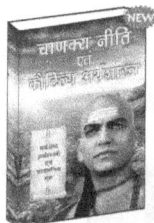

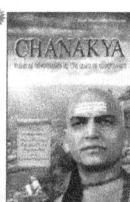

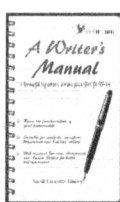

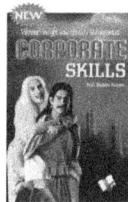

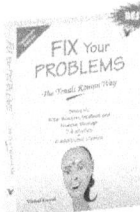

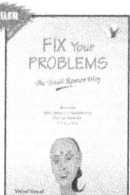

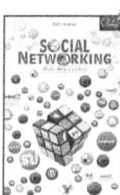

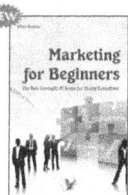

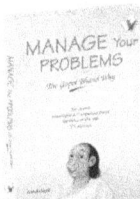

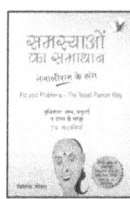

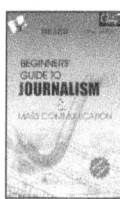

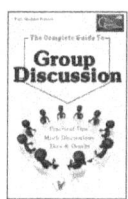

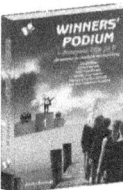

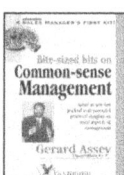

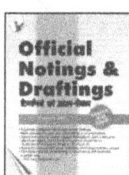

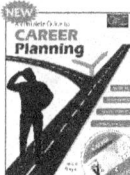

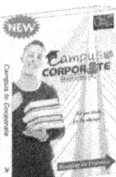

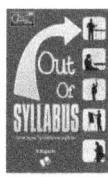

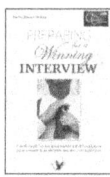

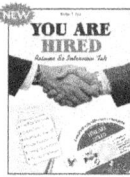

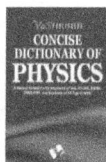

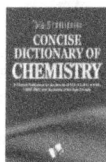

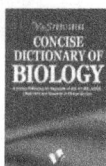

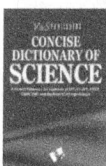

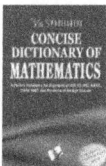

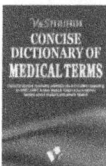

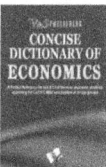

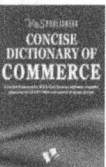

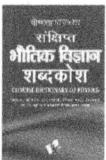

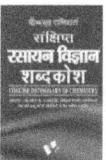

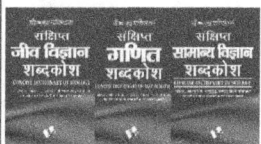

www.ingramcontent.com/pod-product-compliance
Lightning Source LLC
Chambersburg PA
CBHW072222270326
41930CB00010B/1953

* 9 7 8 9 3 5 0 5 7 1 6 6 8 *